Susan Jung

Viral Interference of GB Virus C and Human Immunodeficiency Viruses

Susan Jung

# Viral Interference of GB Virus C and Human Immunodeficiency Viruses

Different GB Virus C Proteins interfere with the Replication of HIV-1

Südwestdeutscher Verlag für Hochschulschriften

**Impressum/Imprint (nur für Deutschland/ only for Germany)**
Bibliografische Information der Deutschen Nationalbibliothek: Die Deutsche Nationalbibliothek verzeichnet diese Publikation in der Deutschen Nationalbibliografie; detaillierte bibliografische Daten sind im Internet über http://dnb.d-nb.de abrufbar.

Alle in diesem Buch genannten Marken und Produktnamen unterliegen warenzeichen-, marken- oder patentrechtlichem Schutz bzw. sind Warenzeichen oder eingetragene Warenzeichen der jeweiligen Inhaber. Die Wiedergabe von Marken, Produktnamen, Gebrauchsnamen, Handelsnamen, Warenbezeichnungen u.s.w. in diesem Werk berechtigt auch ohne besondere Kennzeichnung nicht zu der Annahme, dass solche Namen im Sinne der Warenzeichen- und Markenschutzgesetzgebung als frei zu betrachten wären und daher von jedermann benutzt werden dürften.

Verlag: Südwestdeutscher Verlag für Hochschulschriften GmbH & Co. KG
Dudweiler Landstr. 99, 66123 Saarbrücken, Deutschland
Telefon +49 681 37 20 271-1, Telefax +49 681 37 20 271-0
Email: info@svh-verlag.de
Zugl.: Erlangen, Friedrich-Alexander University Erlangen-Nuremberg, Diss., 2010

Herstellung in Deutschland:
Schaltungsdienst Lange o.H.G., Berlin
Books on Demand GmbH, Norderstedt
Reha GmbH, Saarbrücken
Amazon Distribution GmbH, Leipzig
ISBN: 978-3-8381-2383-7

**Imprint (only for USA, GB)**
Bibliographic information published by the Deutsche Nationalbibliothek: The Deutsche Nationalbibliothek lists this publication in the Deutsche Nationalbibliografie; detailed bibliographic data are available in the Internet at http://dnb.d-nb.de.

Any brand names and product names mentioned in this book are subject to trademark, brand or patent protection and are trademarks or registered trademarks of their respective holders. The use of brand names, product names, common names, trade names, product descriptions etc. even without a particular marking in this works is in no way to be construed to mean that such names may be regarded as unrestricted in respect of trademark and brand protection legislation and could thus be used by anyone.

Publisher: Südwestdeutscher Verlag für Hochschulschriften GmbH & Co. KG
Dudweiler Landstr. 99, 66123 Saarbrücken, Germany
Phone +49 681 37 20 271-1, Fax +49 681 37 20 271-0
Email: info@svh-verlag.de

Printed in the U.S.A.
Printed in the U.K. by (see last page)
ISBN: 978-3-8381-2383-7

Copyright © 2011 by the author and Südwestdeutscher Verlag für Hochschulschriften GmbH & Co. KG and licensors
All rights reserved. Saarbrücken 2011

*To my parents,*

*for their continued support and encouragement.*

# Contents

1. Abstract .................................................................................................. 1
2. Zusammenfassung ................................................................................ 2
3. Introduction ......................................................................................... 3
   3.1. Human Immunodeficiency Virus, the etiologic Agent of AIDS ........ 3
      3.1.1. Structure and Genome Organization .............................................. 4
      3.1.2. Replication ........................................................................................ 5
      3.1.3. Transmission, Prevalence, and Etiopathology ................................ 6

   3.2. GB Virus C, a Pathogen without a Disease ........................................ 8
      3.2.1. Structure and Genome Organization .............................................. 9
      3.2.2. Replication ...................................................................................... 10
      3.2.3. Transmission, Prevalence, and Etiopathology .............................. 10

4. Aims .................................................................................................. 13
5. Results ............................................................................................... 15
   5.1. A Cell Culture System for GB Virus C .............................................. 15
      5.1.1. A Real-Time RT-PCR to detect GB Virus C RNA ........................ 15
      5.1.2. Limited Replication of GB Virus C in Human B and T Cell Lines ... 17
      5.1.3. Increased Replication of GB Virus C in Human Lymphocytes ...... 18

   5.2. Variability of Clinical GB Virus C Isolates ........................................ 20
      5.2.1. A GB Virus C Sera Bank ................................................................ 20
      5.2.2. Differences in the Replication Capacity of Clinical GB Virus C Isolates ... 20
      5.2.3. Sequence Divergence of Clinical GB Virus C Isolates .................. 21

   5.3. Interference of GB Virus C with Human Immunodeficiency Virus ..... 22
      5.3.1. Classification of Clinical GB Virus C Isolates as HIV-Inhibitory and HIV-Non-Inhibitory ... 22
      5.3.2. HIV Impairment by Expression of GB Virus C Gene Cassettes in a Rhadinovirus Vector System ... 26
      5.3.3 Inhibition of different HIV Replication Steps by GB Virus C Proteins ... 27

   5.4. Identification of the GB Virus C E2 Protein as HIV Entry Inhibitor ... 29
      5.4.1. HIV Suppression by Transfection of RNA encoding the GB Virus C Glycoproteins ... 29
      5.4.2. Expression, Purification, and Characterization of GB Virus C E2(340)-Fc Fusion Proteins ... 30
      5.4.3. Mechanism of GB Virus C E2-mediated HIV Inhibition ............... 35

   5.5. Induction of HIV-neutralizing Antibodies by GB Virus C ................ 37
      5.5.1. Screening for anti-E2 Antibodies Positive Blood Donors ............. 37
      5.5.2. HIV Neutralization by anti-E2 Antibodies .................................... 39
      5.5.3. Mechanism of HIV Inhibition by anti-E2 Antibodies ................... 42

6. Discussion ......................................................................................... 47
   6.1. Effect of GB Virus C on HIV in Cell Culture .................................... 47
      6.1.1. Replication Capacity of Clinical of GB Virus C Isolates ............... 47
      6.1.2. Inhibition of HIV Replication by Clinical GB Virus C Isolates ..... 48
      6.1.3. Induction of beta-Chemokines by Clinical GB Virus C Isolates ... 49

| | | | |
|---|---|---|---|
| | 6.2. | Interference of GB Virus C Proteins with HIV Replication | 50 |
| | | 6.2.1. Generation of Human T Cell Lines Expressing GB Virus C Proteins | 50 |
| | | 6.2.2. Suppression of HIV Replication by Several GB Virus C Proteins | 50 |
| | | 6.2.3. Inhibition of HIV Entry by the GB Virus C E2 Protein | 52 |
| | 6.3. | Impairment of HIV Infectivity by anti-E2 Antibodies | 53 |
| 7. | **Methods** | | **57** |
| | 7.1. | Escherichia coli | 57 |
| | | 7.1.1. Preparation of Chemically Competent *E. coli* | 57 |
| | | 7.1.2. Transformation of Chemically Competent *E. coli* | 57 |
| | 7.2. | Preparation, Enzymatic Manipulation, and Analysis of DNA | 58 |
| | | 7.2.1. Purification of DNA | 58 |
| | | 7.2.2. Modification of DNA | 59 |
| | | 7.2.3. Sequencing of DNA | 60 |
| | 7.3. | Preparation, Enzymatic Manipulation, and Analysis of RNA | 60 |
| | | 7.3.1. *In Vitro* Transcription of RNA | 60 |
| | | 7.3.2. Isolation of RNA | 61 |
| | | 7.3.3. Synthesis of cDNA | 61 |
| | 7.4. | Mammalian Cell Culture | 61 |
| | | 7.4.1. Isolation of Peripheral and Cord Blood Mononucleated Cells | 61 |
| | | 7.4.2. Cultivation of Primary Cells and Cell Lines | 62 |
| | | 7.4.3. Cell Proliferation Assay | 62 |
| | | 7.4.4. Long-term Storage of Eukaryotic Cells | 62 |
| | 7.5. | Transfection of DNA and RNA | 62 |
| | | 7.5.1. Calcium Phosphate Transfection | 62 |
| | | 7.5.2. Electroporation | 64 |
| | | 7.5.3. Selection of Eukaryotic Cells | 64 |
| | 7.6. | Expression, Purification, and Analysis of Proteins | 64 |
| | | 7.6.1. Protein Expression in Eukaryotic Cells | 64 |
| | | 7.6.2. Detection of Proteins | 65 |
| | | 7.6.3. Determination of Protein Concentrations | 66 |
| | | 7.6.4. Purification of Proteins by Affinity Chromatography | 67 |
| | | 7.6.5. Deglycosylation of Proteins | 68 |
| | 7.7. | Incubation Assays | 68 |
| | | 7.7.1. Incubation of Human T Cells with GBV-C E2-Fc Fusion Proteins | 68 |
| | | 7.7.2. Incubation of HIV-1 Pseudoparticles with anti-E2 Antibodies | 68 |
| | | 7.7.3. $IC_{50}$ | 68 |
| | 7.8. | Infection Assays | 69 |
| | | 7.8.1. GBV-C Infection of Primary Cells and Cell Lines | 69 |
| | | 7.8.2. Gene Transfer into Human T Cells by *Herpesvirus saimiri* | 69 |
| | | 7.8.3. HIV-1 Infection Assays | 70 |
| | | 7.8.4. Plaque Assays | 71 |

|  |  |  |  |
|---|---|---|---|
| 7.9. | Immuno Assays | | 71 |
| | 7.9.1. | Detection of anti-E2 Antibodies | 71 |
| | 7.9.2. | Detection of Viral and Recombinant GBV-C E2 Proteins | 71 |
| | 7.9.3. | Detection of HIV-1 specific Antibodies | 72 |
| | 7.9.4. | Quantification of HIV p24 | 72 |
| | 7.9.5. | Membrane Lipid Array | 72 |
| 7.10. | Immunohistochemistry | | 72 |
| | 7.10.1. | Immunofluorescence | 72 |
| | 7.10.2. | Flow Cytometry | 72 |
| | 7.10.3. | Fluorescence Activated Cell Sorting | 72 |
| 7.11. | Polymerase Chain Reactions | | 73 |
| | 7.11.1. | Molecular Cloning of Recombinant Proteins | 73 |
| | 7.11.2. | Colony PCR | 73 |
| | 7.11.3. | Quantification of Viral DNA by Real-Time PCR | 73 |
| | 7.11.4. | Quantification of Viral RNA by Real-Time RT-PCR | 74 |

8. **Material** .................................................................................................. 77

    8.1. Media, Buffers, and Solutions    77
        8.1.1. Media, Buffers, and Solutions for Prokaryotic Cell Culture    77
        8.1.2. Media, Buffers, and Solutions for Eukaryotic Cell Culture    77
        8.1.3. Media, Buffers, and Solutions for Protein Analysis    79

    8.2. Cells    81
        8.2.1. *Escherichia coli*    81
        8.2.2. Mammalian Cell Lines    82

    8.3. Antibodies and Normal Sera    83

    8.4. Plasmids    84
        8.4.1. GBV-C Expression Plasmids    84
        8.4.2. HIV Expression Plasmids    86
        8.4.3. Other Expression Constructs    87

    8.5. Oligonucleotides    88
        8.5.1. GBV-C specific Primers and Probes    88
        8.5.2. Other Gene specific Primers and Probes    90

    8.6. Kits and Enzymes    90
    8.7. Chemicals    91
    8.8. Consumables    93

9. **Abbreviations** ........................................................................................ 95
10. **Bibliography** ........................................................................................... 97
11. **Publications** ......................................................................................... 104
13. **Acknowledgements** ........................................................................... 105

# List of Figures

Figure 3-1: Structure of an HIV particle. ...................................................................................................4
Figure 3-2: HIV replication cycle. ...........................................................................................................5
Figure 3-3: Unrooted phylogenetic tree of various members of the *Flaviviridae*. ................................9
Figure 3-4: Seroprevalence of GBV-C. ..................................................................................................11
Figure 5-1: Comparison of different RNA purification methods. ......................................................15
Figure 5-2: Detection of GBV-C RNA using the AbiPrism® 7700 and 7000. .................................16
Figure 5-3: Replication of GBV-C on human B and T cell lines. .....................................................17
Figure 5-4: Replication of GBV-C on PBMC. ....................................................................................18
Figure 5-5: Replication of GBV-C on CBL. ........................................................................................19
Figure 5-6: Correlation of GBV-C virus load and HIV status. ..........................................................20
Figure 5-7: Variability of the replication capacity of clinical GBV-C isolates. .................................21
Figure 5-8: Mutations in the amino acid sequence of the envelope protein E2 of clinical GBV-C isolates. .....22
Figure 5-9: Clinical GBV-C isolates differ in their HIV-inhibitory phenotype. ..............................23
Figure 5-10: Inhibition of $HIV_{WT}$ by purified GBV-C virions. ........................................................23
Figure 5-11: Inhibition of $HIV_{PP}$ by clinical GBV-C isolates. .........................................................24
Figure 5-12: Down regulation of CCR5 surface expression by HIV-inhibitory GBV-C isolates. ..........25
Figure 5-13: Chemokine induction by HIV-inhibitory GBV-C isolates. ...........................................25
Figure 5-14: Generation of T cell lines stable expressing different GBV-C genes by infection of $HVS_{GBV-C}$. .....26
Figure 5-15: Protein expression in $HVS_{GBV-C}$ transformed T cell lines. ...........................................27
Figure 5-16: HIV inhibition on $HVS_{GBV-C}$ transformed T cell lines. ...............................................27
Figure 5-17: Vectors for eukaryotic expression of GBV-C proteins. ..................................................28
Figure 5-18: Expression of GBV-C proteins in CEMx174$_{CCR5}$ Tet-Off cells. ..................................28
Figure 5-19: Inhibition of $HIV_{PP}$ by the GBV-C proteins E2, NS3, and NS5A. ............................29
Figure 5-20: Inhibition of $HIV_{WT}$ by transfection of RNA encoding the GBV-C envelope proteins. .......30
Figure 5-21: Model of the GBV-C envelope proteins E1 and E2. ....................................................31
Figure 5-22: Expression of GBV-C E2(340)-Fc fusion proteins in 293T cells. ................................32
Figure 5-23: Characterization of Fc fusion proteins. ...........................................................................32
Figure 5-24: Inhibition of $HIV_{WT}$ and $HIV_{PP}$ by recombinant GBV-C E2 proteins. .......................33
Figure 5-25: E2(340)-Fc fusion proteins inhibit the gp120/CD4-dependent HIV entry mechanism. .....34
Figure 5-26: Down regulation of CCR5 surface expression by recombinant GBV-C E2 proteins. ......35
Figure 5-27: Chemokine and cytokine induction by recombinant GBV-C E2 proteins. ................36
Figure 5-28: Recombinant GBV-C E2 proteins bind to human cells. ...............................................37
Figure 5-29: Screening for GBV-C anti-E2 antibodies. .......................................................................38
Figure 5-30: Determent of the IgG isotype of human anti-E2 antibodies. .......................................39
Figure 5-31: Neutralization of $HIV_{WT}$ by anti-E2 antibodies. ..........................................................40
Figure 5-32: Neutralization of $HIV_{PP}$ by anti-E2 antibodies. ...........................................................41
Figure 5-33: Neutralization ability of anti-E2 antibodies is restricted to HIV. .................................42
Figure 5-34: Neutralization of the anti-E2 antibodies mediated HIV-inhibitory effect. ................43
Figure 5-35: Immunoprecipitation of $HIV_{PP}$ by anti-E2 antibodies. ................................................43
Figure 5-36: Cell binding by anti-E2 antibodies. ..................................................................................44
Figure 5-37: Binding of anti-E2 antibodies to phosphatidylinositols. ................................................45
Figure 7-1: Calculation of the transformation efficiency. ....................................................................57
Figure 7-2: Calculation of picomoles of DNA ends. ..........................................................................59
Figure 7-3: Calculation of micrograms to picomoles of DNA. .........................................................60
Figure 7-4: pH range of different electrophoresis buffers. .................................................................66
Figure 7-5: Cytopathic effect of *Herpesvirus saimiri* on OMK cells. ..................................................70
Figure 7-6: Calculation of the $TCID_{50}$. ................................................................................................71

# List of Tables

| | | |
|---|---|---|
| Table 7-1: | Conditions for agarose gel electrophoresis. | 58 |
| Table 7-2: | Amount of template DNA and cycle condition for standard DNA sequencing. | 60 |
| Table 7-3: | Recipes for transfection mixtures prepared in HeBS. | 63 |
| Table 7-4: | Recipes for transfection mixtures prepared in BES. | 63 |
| Table 7-5: | Recipes for BES-based HIV$_{PP}$ production. | 63 |
| Table 7-6: | Selection conditions for 293T and CEMx174$_{CCR5}$ cells. | 64 |
| Table 7-7: | Recipes for denaturing polyacrylamide separating and stacking gels. | 65 |
| Table 7-8: | Amplification characteristics of selected proteins for high fidelity PCR. | 73 |
| Table 7-9: | Reaction mix and thermal cycle conditions for colony PCR. | 73 |
| Table 7-10: | Reaction mix and thermal cycle conditions to quantify Adenovirus DNA. | 74 |
| Table 7-11: | Reaction mix and thermal cycle conditions to quantify *Herpesvirus saimiri* DNA. | 74 |
| Table 7-12: | Reaction mix and thermal cycle conditions to quantify YFV RNA. | 74 |
| Table 7-13: | Reaction mix and thermal cycle conditions to quantify GBV-C RNA (ThermoScript). | 75 |
| Table 7-14: | Reaction mix and thermal cycle conditions to quantify GBV-C RNA (SuperScript III). | 75 |
| Table 8-1: | Antibiotics for prokaryotic selection. | 77 |
| Table 8-2: | Preparation of potassium phosphate buffer at 25°C. | 80 |
| Table 8-3: | Preparation of sodium phosphate buffer at 25°C. | 81 |

# 1. Abstract

GB Virus C (GBV-C) was discovered in 1995 within the search for new hepatitis viruses. The human apathogenic enveloped RNA virus belongs to the family of the *Flaviviridae* and replicates primarily in lymphocytes. Transmission occurs mainly by sexual or parenteral exposure. In developed countries up to 6% of the healthy population and up to 40% of multiply exposed individuals, such as HIV patients, are viremic for GBV-C. Since the late 1990s, GBV-C has been investigated in the context of HIV. Unexpectedly, epidemiological studies demonstrate that GBV-C infection is not associated with faster progression of HIV disease. Remarkably, long-term GBV-C viremia correlates with a better clinical outcome of HIV disease leading to improved survival of GBV-C/HIV co-infected patients. However, epidemiological studies cannot prove a causal relationship nor they distinguish whether the positive impact of GBV-C on HIV mortality is caused by direct viral interference of GBV-C and HIV or if GBV-C serves just as a surrogate marker for a robust immune system or an unidentified factor. In the present study, the interference of GBV-C and HIV was investigated in cell culture experiments. After a GBV-C sera bank was built up and a suitable GBV-C replication system could be established, several GBV-C isolates were characterized in GBV-C/HIV co-infection experiments. GBV-C infection as well as transfection of GBV-C RNA mediated a strong inhibition of several CCR5- and CXCR4-tropic HIV strains and clades. Interestingly, clinical GBV-C isolates differed in their ability to inhibit HIV and were classified according their HIV-inhibitory phenotype as HIV-inhibitory or HIV-non-inhibitory GBV-C isolates. Thereby, the inhibitory effect did not depend on GBV-C replication and was mediated, at least in part, by induction of beta-chemokines and down regulation of CCR5 on the cell surface. Further co-infection assays implied that GBV-C affects different HIV replication steps and that several GBV-C proteins may be involved in efficient HIV suppression. Indeed, protein-screening assays identified three GBV-C proteins with HIV-inhibitory capacity. Whereas the GBV-C glycoprotein E2 inhibited exclusively the gp120/CD4 mediated cell entry of HIV, the nonstructural GBV-C proteins NS3 and NS5A impaired later steps of HIV replication. Recombinant E2(340)-Fc fusion proteins derived from clinical GBV-C isolates corroborated the HIV-entry inhibitory ability of the GBV-C E2 protein as well as the existence of various HIV-inhibitory phenotypes of clinical GBV-C isolates. In addition to the GBV-C E2 protein, also antibodies elicited by the GBV-C E2 protein mediated efficient neutralization of HIV replication. Thereby, HIV-neutralizing anti-E2 antibodies cross reacted with HIV virions independent of the HIV glycoprotein gp120. Comparable to the broad reactive human anti-gp41 antibodies 2F5 and 4E10, HIV-neutralizing anti-E2 antibodies bound to phosphatidylinositol-4-phosphate (PI(4)P) within the virus lipid bilayer. In summary, GBV-C proteins as well as anti-E2 antibodies seem to be responsible for the beneficial effect of GBV-C on HIV in co-infected patients. Most notably, a combination of the inhibitory effects of the GBV-C E2 protein and of HIV-neutralizing anti-E2 antibodies presents an innovative approach for further drug development and/or vaccine design.

## 2. Zusammenfassung

Das GB Virus-C (GBV-C) wurde 1995 im Rahmen der Suche nach neuen Hepatitisviren entdeckt. Das humane, apathogene, umhüllte RNA-Virus gehört zur Familie der *Flaviviridae* und repliziert überwiegend in B- und T-Lymphozyten. Die Übertragung erfolgt hauptsächlich sexuell oder parenteral. In Industrieländern sind bis zu 6% der gesunden Bevölkerung und bis zu 40% der Personen aus Risikokollektiven, z. Bsp. HIV-Patienten, virämisch. Seit den späten 1990ern wurde daher der Einfluss von GBV-C auf den Verlauf der HIV-Erkrankung genauer untersucht. Entgegen den Erwartungen zeigten die klinischen Studien aber, dass die GBV-C-Koinfektion nicht mit einer schnelleren HIV-Progression korreliert. Im Gegenteil, besonders die chronische GBV-C-Infektion ist mit einem besseren HIV-Krankheitsverlauf und einer höheren Überlebenswahrscheinlichkeit GBV-C/HIV-koinfizierter Patienten assoziiert. Klinische Studien beweisen aber keinen kausalen Zusammenhang und können nicht differenzieren, ob der beobachtete Einfluss von GBV-C auf die HIV-Mortalität durch die virale Interferenz von GBV-C und HIV bedingt ist, oder ob GBV-C nur einen Surrogatmarker für ein robustes Immunsystem oder einen unbekannten Faktor darstellt. Im Rahmen dieser Arbeit wurde daher die Interferenz von GBV-C und HIV in Zellkulturexperimenten untersucht. Nach dem Aufbau einer Serumbank und der Etablierung eines Replikationssystems für GBV-C, wurden klinische GBV-C-Isolate in GBV-C/HIV-Koinfektionsversuchen charakterisiert. Sowohl durch Infektion mit GBV-C, als auch durch Transfektion von GBV-C-kodierender RNA konnte eine starke Inhibition verschiedener CCR5- und CXCR4-tropher HIV-Subtypen induziert werden. Interessanterweise unterschieden sich die klinischen GBV-C-Isolate in ihrer Fähigkeit die HIV-Replikation zu supprimieren und konnten anhand ihres HIV-inhibitorischen Phänotyps als HIV-inhibitorisch und nicht-HIV-inhibitorisch klassifiziert werden. Der HIV-inhibitorische Effekt war unabhängig von der GBV-C-Replikation und war zumindest teilweise durch die Induktion von beta-Chemokinen und eine reduzierte CCR5-Oberflächenexpression verursacht. Weitere Experimente zeigten, dass unterschiedliche HIV-Replikationsschritte durch verschiedene GBV-C-Proteine gehemmt werden. Insgesamt wurden drei HIV-inhibitorische GBV-C-Proteine identifiziert. Während das E2-Protein den gp120/CD4 vermittelten HIV-Zelleintritt inhibierte, supprimierten das NS3- und NS5A-Protein spätere Replikationsschritte von HIV. Durch rekombinante E2(340)-Fc-Fusionsproteine konnte sowohl die hemmende Wirkung des GBV-C-E2-Glykoproteins als auch die Existenz unterschiedlicher HIV-inhibitorischen Phänotypen klinischer GBV-C Isolate untermauert werden. Neben dem GBV-C-E2-Protein vermitteln auch Antikörper, die gegen das GBV-C-E2-Protein gerichtet sind eine Hemmung der HIV-Replikation. Unabhängig vom HIV-Oberflächenprotein gp120 kreuzreagieren HIV-neutralisierende Anti-E2-Antikörper mit HIV-Partikeln. Vergleichbar mit den humanen, breit-wirksamen, HIV-neutralisierenden Anti-gp41-Antikörpern 2F5 und 4E10, binden diese Anti-E2-Antikörper an Phosphatidyl-Inositol-4-Phosphat (PI(4)P) in der Virusmembran. Zusammenfassend scheinen für den positiven Effekt von GBV-C auf HIV in koinfizierten Patienten mehrere GBV-C-Proteine und Anti-E2-Antikörper verantwortlich zu sein. Die Kombination der HIV-inhibitorischen Effekte des E2-Proteins und der HIV-neutralisierenden Anti-E2-Antikörper stellt dabei einen innovativen Ansatz für zukünftige Medikamentenentwicklungen und/oder das Impfstoffdesign dar.

# 3. Introduction

Simultaneous infection by two or more pathogens are not uncommon and each individual virus can provide and profit from synergistic contributions by direct interactions such as genetic recombination, functional complementation, or reduced immune response. Co-infection of a host by multiple pathogens has important epidemiological and clinical implications. However, the direction and magnitude of effects vary considerably. In conjunction with human immunodeficiency virus (HIV), co-infections are associated with a significantly decreased survival probability[202]. Particularly, hepatitis co-infection and notably chronic hepatitis C virus (HCV) co-infection affecting 25% of HIV positive patients[31,285], accelerates the progression of HIV infection to the acquired immunodeficiency syndrome (AIDS)[31,78,202,297]. HCV-related liver diseases have emerged as the most clinically relevant co-morbidities in the HIV-infected population[29,275]. In contrast, only a few coincident infections, such as scrub typhus, human herpesvirus 6, influenza A virus, measles, and dengue virus can result in suppression of HIV replication[110,185,222,238,303]. Thereby, the HIV-inhibitory effect is transient and limited to cell culture experiments. Considering this background, it was surprisingly that GB Virus C (GBV-C) co-infection leads to contrary effects in GBV-C/HIV co-infected patients. GBV-C is assumed to be an apathogenic, blood born virus. In untreated HIV patients, long-term GBV-C viremia is associated with a better clinical outcome of HIV disease progression as compared to HIV positive patients, who are GBV-C negative. The observed beneficial effects include higher CD4 baselines and a slower decline in CD4 T cell counts as well as lower HIV viremia in plasma, decreased need for antiretroviral therapy (ART), decreased mortality, improved AIDS-free survival rates, and a significantly smaller increase in HIV RNA concentration during the first five to six years following HIV seroconversion[287,317]. Although some epidemiological studies could not support these beneficial effects[24,28,38], no studies have been published reporting a negative outcome of GBV-C co-infection. Therefore, the beneficial role for GBV-C in HIV positive patients is widely accepted and understanding the mechanisms of GBV-C/HIV interference may identify novel approaches for HIV therapy.

## 3.1. Human Immunodeficiency Virus, the etiologic Agent of AIDS

In the late 1970s and early 1980s, the US Centers for Disease Control and Prevention reported about a cluster of previously healthy patients with symptoms of a defect in cell-mediated immunity[42,43]. In 1983, scientists at the Pasteur Institute isolated an agent from the lymph node of an individual with generalized lymphadenopathy of unknown origin[189]. The associated virus was cytopathic in human peripheral blood mononucleated cells (PBMC) specifically killing the subset of CD4 positive T lymphocytes, and released high titers of progeny virions. The virions contained reverse transcriptase activity and exhibited morphologic and genetic features that were typical for retroviruses[14,94]. This new retrovirus, which is associated with AIDS, was named human immunodeficiency virus type 1 (HIV-1) and was found in the United States, Europe, and central Africa[55]. In 1986, a related, but less pathogenic human retrovirus, named HIV-2, has been found mainly in infected individuals in western Africa[53]. HIV-1 isolates are classified into group M (major), group O (outlier), and group N (non-M/non-O). Group M can be further subdivided into nine subtypes or clades (A to K) as well as several recombinant isolates. HIV is widely distributed and sub-subtypes and recombinant forms have emerged over the past decades[182,183,218,235]. Although subtype B is predominant in North America, Western Europe, and Australia, subtype A and C are responsible for the majority of HIV cases in the worldwide epidemic[206,326]. Except recombinant HIV-1 isolates, there are clear evidences that HIV types and subtypes have arisen through cross-species transmission from nonhuman primates in Africa. Phylogenic analyses indicate that HIV-1 and HIV-2 have distinct origins[96,124,127,258,259].

### 3.1.1. Structure and Genome Organization

Electron microscopic analyses revealed 100–120µm enveloped virions that are surrounded by a lipoprotein-rich membrane. HIV particles contain a cone-shaped cylindrical core composed of 2000 copies of the viral capsid protein p24$^{CA}$ enclosing a diploid, single-stranded RNA genome that is coated with the nucleocapsid protein p7$^{NC}$. The two RNA genomes are about 9.7kb and present as a dimer. The conical core contains the viral enzymes required for early replication events (reverse transcriptase, p51$^{RT}$ and p66$^{RT}$; integrase, p32$^{IN}$). In addition to the conical capsid, the inner portion of the viral membrane contains the viral protease p10$^{PR}$. It is surrounded by the myristoylated matrix protein p17$^{MA}$, which is anchored to the inside of the viral lipid membrane. The envelope proteins are derived from a gp160 precursor glycoprotein that is cleaved into a gp41$^{TM}$ transmembrane and a heavily glycosylated gp120$^{SU}$ surface protein. The two proteins form an average of ten gp41-gp120 trimers as well as up to hundred tufts made up of trimeric gp41 with various numbers of gp120 monomers on the virion surface[76,98,99,103,104,152,181,307,324,325]. During the HIV budding process from specific lipid domains, virions incorporate different host cell proteins, such as histocompatibility leukocyte antigens (HLA) class I and II, cell adhesion surface proteins, cytoskeletal proteins, cyclophilin A, and ubiquitin[6,207,208]. In addition to the structural proteins, the virus contains also regulatory (Tat, Rev) and accessory proteins (Nef, Vif, Vpu, Vpr), which play key roles in modulating virus replication. The RNA binding proteins Tat and Rev are expressed early in the viral life cycle and are essential for viral replication. Whereas Tat promotes the transcription of HIV genes, Rev ensures the export of correctly processed messenger and genomic RNA from the nucleus to the cytoplasma[79,108,266]. Nef has multiple functions including cell activation due to cellular signal transduction as well as down regulation of CD4 on the cell surface[246]. Vif enhances the infectiveness of progeny virus particles. Vpu is necessary for virus assembly and virus budding. Vpr is involved in the arrest of the cell cycle and enables reverse transcribed DNA to gain access to the nucleus in non-dividing cells[108]. Whereas Nef and Vif are closely associated with the core, Vpu is found most likely outside the core. Vpr could be detected in virions and cells as well as in sera and cerebrospinal fluids of AIDS patients indicating that it exerts its biological functions via different mechanisms[40,156,165, 169,213]. The genomic size of HIV is about 10kb with three overlapping open reading frames (ORF)

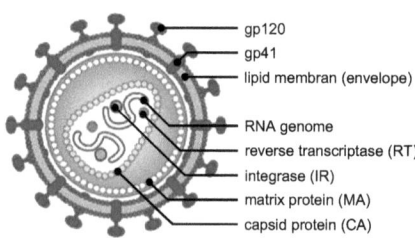

**Figure 3-1: Structure of an HIV particle.** From www.roshanpakistan.com with modifications.

coding for several viral proteins. The genome is characterized by the presence of the genes *gag*, *pol*, and *env*, which code the primary translation products p55$^{Gag}$ (Gag precursor), p160$^{Gag-Pol}$ (Gag/Pol precursor), and gp160$^{Env}$ (Env precursor). The precursor p55$^{Gag}$ contains the structural proteins of the core (CA, NC, p6) as well as the matrix protein. The p160$^{Gag-Pol}$ precursor polyprotein is a fusion between the Gag and Pol polyprotein and is translated as the result of a -1 translational frameshift. Several p160$^{Gag-Pol}$ precursor polyproteins are packaged into the assembling virion. Without assistance from cellular proteases, processing of p160$^{Gag-Pol}$ is accomplished by the viral protease encoded within the Gag-Pol precursor. Cleavage gives rise to the protease, the reverse transcriptase, and the integrase. The glycosylated Env precursor is converted by the endoprotease furin into the viral envelope glycoproteins gp120 and gp41[56,60,90,113,271].

## 3.1.2. Replication

The initial event in HIV infection is binding of the envelope glycoprotein to the CD4 receptor present on the surface of CD4 positive cells of the immune system including T lymphocytes, macrophages, and dendritic cells. HIV cell entry involves the formation of a tri-molecular complex among the gp120, the primary receptor CD4, and the chemokine receptor CCR5 or CXCR4. Upon binding of gp120 to CD4 and interaction with the respective co-receptor, conformational changes in gp120 and gp41 occur. The gp41 ectodomain adopts an extended conformation and the N-terminal fusion peptide inserts into the lipid bilayer of the target cell. The N- and C-helices of the gp41 ectodomain undergoes rearrangements and fold into a six-helix bundle that brings cellular and viral bilayer in apposition and membrane fusion takes

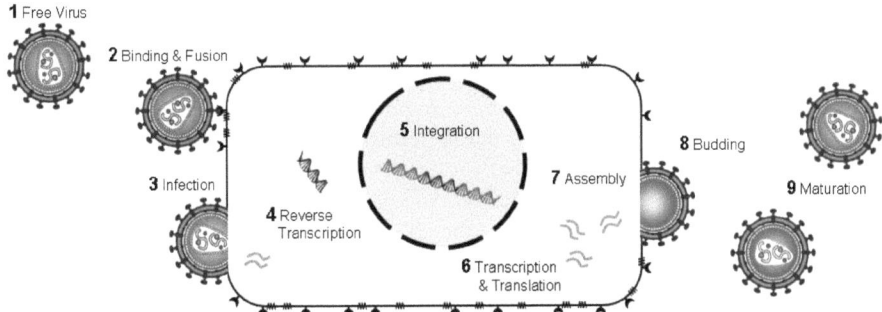

**Figure 3-2: HIV replication cycle.** Free virus (1) binds tightly by its gp120 glycoprotein to a CD4 molecule on the cell surface. The binding of gp120 to CD4 results in a conformational change in the gp120 molecule allowing it to bind to a co-receptor (either CCR5 or CXCR4). After virus adsorption, viral envelope and cell membrane fuse together (2) and the viral core is released into the cytoplasm (3), where the virion-associated reverse transcriptase is activated and begins to convert single stands of viral RNA into double-stranded DNA (4). The newly made HIV DNA is transported to the nucleus, where it is integrated into the host cell genome with the help of the HIV integrase (5). Controlled by viral gene products as well as the cellular machinery, transcription of integrated viral cDNA leads to the production of genomic (unspliced) and messenger (spliced) RNA (mRNA) molecules that are transported to the cell cytoplasm, where the virus co-opts the cellular protein-making machinery. Translation of HIV mRNA leads to the production of Env proteins and immature precursors of capsid (Gag) and viral polymerase (Pol) proteins (6). Immature Gag and fused Gag-Pol precursors are transported to the cell membrane, where the viral progeny begins assembling (7) and buds off from the infected cell acquiring an envelope that includes both cellular and viral proteins from the cell membrane (8). Viral particles released following budding, however, do not contain the characteristic condensed core and are not yet infectious. Gag and Pol precursor proteins that built up the immature viral core are cleaved by the viral protease into smaller functional polypeptides. This step results in infectious virions (9).

place. The viral core gains entry into the host cell cytoplasma and the outer lipid enveloped is removed. The reverse transcription complex is formed and reverse transcription of the viral RNA genome into double-stranded cDNA is mediated by minus-strand polymerization due to the ribonuclease (RNase) H active site of the RT. When the viral RNA is transcribed into a RNA/DNA hybrid, the RNase H activity of the RT breaks down the RNA stand. The polymerase active site of the RT completes the complementary DNA strand forming a double-stranded DNA molecule. The proviral cDNA associates with MA, IN, and Vpr and forms the preintegration complex that is translocated to the nucleus. Although circular and linear forms of proviral cDNA exist, the IN catalyzes exclusively integration of linear double-stranded cDNA within the host cell genome. Therefore, the IN clips off several nucleotides from the 3' terminis creating two sticky 3'-recessed ends, transfers the modified provirus DNA into the cell nucleus, and makes a staggered cleavage in the cellular target DNA to join the 3'-recessed ends of viral and cellular DNA prior cellular repair enzymes fill the gaps. Integration of the HIV provirus marks the end of the initial phase of the HIV life cycle, which is driven by viral enzymes. Upon cell activation and driven by host factors, transcription and translation of viral RNA and HIV proteins occurs. Initially, regulatory proteins, such as Tat and Rev, are synthesized. Transcription is stimulated by Tat binding to the transactivation response element and viral messenger RNA migrates into the cytoplasm. Rev facilitates expression of structural and enzymatic genes and inhibits the production of regulatory proteins therefore promoting the formation of mature virus particles. In a stepwise process new virions are formed. Thereby, human immunodeficiency viruses as well as many other enveloped viruses are released from the host cell by budding. Assembly of HIV virions is directed by Gag that coordinates the incorporation of each of the viral components as well as of a number of host cell factors into the assembling particle. Gag and Gag-Pol precursors are transported to the inner leaflet of the plasma membrane and proteins coded by *gag* and *pol* form the nucleus of maturing virions. Two viral RNA molecules associate with replication enzymes, while core proteins assemble over them and from the virus capsid. Env glycoprotein precursors, which are cleaved into the gp120 and gp41 subunits by a host protease during trafficking through the Golgi apparatus, are incorporated in the virus lipid membrane. The virion grows until a roughly spherical particle is finally pinched off and released from the cell. Progeny virions are immature and the large viral precursor molecules have to be cleaved by the HIV protease to form mature, infectious HIV particles. During the budding process through the host cell membrane, the viral membrane becomes enriched with cellular proteins, phospholipids, and cholesterol[61,71,80,90].

## 3.1.3. Transmission, Prevalence, and Etiopathology

HIV is mainly transmitted by contaminated blood, sexual contact, and from mother to child. Thereby, transmission efficiency is greatly influenced by the viral load in the body fluid to which an individual is exposed. The highest virus concentrations are observed in peripheral blood mononucleated cells (PBMC), blood plasma, cerebrospinal fluid, semen, and female genital secretions[39,136,229,260]. Modes of transmission vary in different geographic regions. In the United States, transmission occurs mainly via homosexual contact, whereas heterosexual transmission is most common in large parts of the world outside the United States[112,144,294]. Despite the benefits of antiretroviral therapy (ART), since 2000 the global percentage of adults living with HIV has leveled off. The rate of new infections has fallen in several countries, but globally these favorable trends are at least partially offset by increases in new infections in other countries. The number of people living with HIV worldwide continued to grow in 2008 reaching an estimated 33.4 million. The nine countries with the highest HIV prevalence worldwide are located in the sub-Saharan Africa. With prevalence rates greater than 20% and with 5.7 million HIV infected individuals, South Africa is home to the world's largest population of people living with HIV. In 2008, it is estimated that 2.7 million new HIV infections and 2 million deaths due to AIDS-related illnesses occurred worldwide. Globally, the total number of people living with HIV was more than 20% higher than in 2000, and the prevalence was roughly threefold higher than in 1990. The continuing rise in the population of people living with HIV reflects the combined effects of continued high rates of new HIV infections and the beneficial impact of ART[294].

The course of HIV infection is characterized by different phases. The first ten days after virus transmission, before viral RNA becomes detectable in the blood plasma, are summarized as eclipse phase. During the acute phase, at the end of the eclipse phase, virus and virus-infected cells reach the draining lymph node. HIV replicates rapidly and spreads throughout the body to other lymphoid tissues, particularly gut-associated lymphoid tissues (GALT), where a high number of activated CD4 and CCR5 positive memory T cells are present. Approximately 20% of CD4 positive lymphocytes become infected and 60% of uninfected CD4 T cells in the GALT become activated. Within the first three weeks of HIV infection most of the activated cells die due to apoptosis[35,97]. Plasma viremia increases exponentially and reaches a peak 21 to 28 days after infection. At the point of peak viremia, the initial virus population is relatively homogeneous and generally macrophage-tropic, since the immune response has not yet affected the amino acid sequence of the virus. The CD4 T cell count decreases and is low at the time of peak viremia, but returns later to near normal levels in the blood but not in the GALT[35]. HIV viremia is greatly curtailed within a few weeks after transmission by cell-mediated immune responses as the number of CD8 positive cytotoxic lymphocytes increases before neutralizing antibodies arise approximately 12 weeks after HIV transmission[32,149,214,304]. The degree of viremia at this stage is a direct predictor of HIV progression. In the absence of ART, this set point is maintained by a balance between virus turnover and immune response and it marks the beginning of the asymptomatic stage[220,248]. During the phase of clinical latency, HIV virus load in the blood is low and the virus population becomes more heterogeneous. Under the pressure of adaptive immune responses, virus diversification occurs and escape mutants are established[224]. Finally, the infected individual develops AIDS-related symptoms characterized by a cell count of CD4 positive lymphocytes below 200 per milliliter and increased quantities of virus, which marks the entrance into the symptomatic phase of HIV infection[178]. Due to increased virus replication in lymph nodes and lymphoid cells, the architecture of lymphoid tissues is destroyed. Besides the CD4 T cell count, also the number of CD8 positive cytotoxic lymphocytes decreases. The late-emerging virus population becomes homogeneous again and infects predominantly T lymphocytes. CXCR4-tropic HIV are less sensitive to neutralizing antibodies and more responsive to antibodies, which enhance virus infectivity[86,105,115,198,304]. Strains that have enhanced neurotropism or increased pathogenicity for other organ systems emerge due to specific mutations in the viral envelope or regulatory genes[75,86].

The development of potent antiretroviral agents result in an abundance of treatment option. A number of viral replication steps and enzymes can be targeted: fusion, entry, reverse transcription, integration as well as the protease[65]. Optimal use of highly active antiretroviral therapy (HAART) significantly declines the AIDS-related morbidity and mortality and leads to increased survival of HIV infected individuals[33,230]. Due to the rapid turnover of HIV and the high error rate of the RT, drug-resistance can occur, which is most likely under suboptimal therapy or with low adherence or malabsorption leading to insufficient suppression of viral replication[46,128,142]. However, the majority of HIV infected individuals have just a limited or no access to ART. Furthermore, antiretroviral drugs are associated with a wide spectrum of side effects and not able to eradicate HIV infection. Therefore, the most potent strategy in preventing further spread of the HIV epidemic will be a safe and effective vaccine. Neutralizing antibodies and cytotoxic T cells are the major effectors of anti-viral immunity. Hereby, antibodies are the only component of the adaptive immune response that can neutralize a virus particle prior to infection of a cell. A number of different vaccine candidates such as recombinant envelope or Gag proteins produced in different cell systems, peptides derived from the V3 loop, gag sequences in live recombinant vectors and virus like particles as well as nucleic acid based agents have been evaluated. Even though, none of these approaches were successful to induce sufficient protection against an HIV infection[17,34,41,93,119,141,150,176,241,256,257].

## 3.2. GB Virus C, a Pathogen without a Disease

Despite the discovery of the hepatitis C virus (HCV) in 1989[49], the etiology of a substantial fraction of post-transfusion and community-acquired hepatitis cases has remained undefined [8,9]. In the course of the search for new hepatitis viruses, Deinhardt *et al.* attempted to induce hepatitis in marmosets by inoculation with human serum derived from volunteers exhibiting some of the characteristics of human viral hepatitis. Exclusively marmosets that were inoculated with serum of the 34-year-old surgeon George Barker (GB), who had developed hepatitis of unknown origin, but had not knowingly exposed himself to serum hepatitis, displayed abnormal hepatic tests and liver biopsies. The unknown agent could be serially passaged and specimens of GB and the infected marmosets were stored[1,68]. Subsequent primate host range and cross challenge experiments suggested that the GB agent was distinct from currently known human hepatitis viruses[69,228,276]. In 1995, genomes of two unknown viruses (GB Virus type A, GBV-A; GB Virus type B, GBV-B) were identified in the plasma from a marmoset infected with the GB agent. Sequence analysis indicated limited amino acid concordance of the predicted polyproteins with HCV suggesting that the GB agent contains two unique flavivirus-like genomes[249,264]. Even though, GBV-A and GBV-B turned out to be viruses that are exclusively found in Tamarins, ELISA using recombinant GBV-A and GBV-B proteins as well as RT-PCR using degenerated primers for the helicase region of flaviviruses revealed the presence of a virus-like nucleotide sequence in blood donors that had been tested negative for HCV and HBV. Sequence analysis displayed a high degree of nucleotide (59%) and amino acid sequence similarity (73%). The virus was termed GB virus type C (GBV-C). The GB viruses constituted a separate phylogenic group within the family of the *Flaviviridae*[157,263]. At the same time, another research group identified a cDNA clone from an HCV-infected patient, who was originally identified as having a viral, non-A, non-B hepatitis. The sequence of the virus, termed Hepatitis G virus (HGV), did not match any sequence in the GenBank database and contained one continuous ORF coding for a single polyprotein. Further analysis of the amino acid sequence revealed that HGV and the GB viruses are similar. Comparison with a fragment of the putative NS3 region of GBV-C indicated an 86% nucleotide and a 100% amino acid identity suggesting that HGV and GBV-C are very closely related and that both viruses represent different isolates of the same virus[164]. GBV-C has been shown to exist as a group of six genotypes, which show consistent geographical clustering. Genotype 1 predominates in West Africa, genotype 2 in North and South America as well as in Europe, genotype 3 in Southeast Asia, genotype 4 in Southeast Asia and Japan, genotype 5 in South Africa, and genotype 6

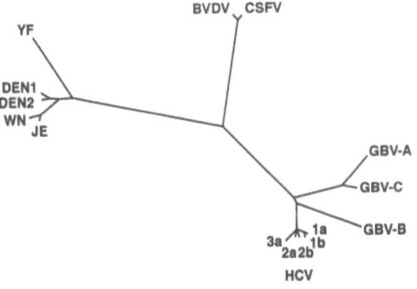

Figure 3-3: Unrooted phylogenetic tree of various members of the Flaviviridae. Amino acid sequences of the GB viruses, representative members of HCV genotypes, the pestiviruses (bovine viral diarrhea virus, BVDV; classical swine fever virus, CSFV), and the flaviviruses (dengue virus type 1 and 2, DEN1 and DEN2; yellow fever virus, YF; West Nile virus, WN; Japanese encephalitis virus, JE) were aligned[261].

is found in Indonesia[194,199,291]. Depending of the genotype, the prevalence of GBV-C RNA in blood donors vary between 2.5% and 13.9%[2,50,72,133,194,200,201,210,245,282,291,293,302]. Although no significant correlation between ethnicity of donors and prevalence of GBV-C viremia could be observed, the prevalence of genotypes 1 and 5 is significant higher than the prevalence of other GBV-C genotypes[309]. GBV-C is more highly conserved than HCV and exhibit only about 11% divergence between genotypes compared to about 30% for HCV[194]. The worldwide geographical distribution of GBV-C variants suggests a long evolutionary history that parallels prehistoric human migration and implies a low mutational rate of this RNA virus[265].

### 3.2.1. Structure and Genome Organization

GBV-C virions appear to be spherical with a diameter of 40–60nm and are composed of a lipid bilayer surrounding the single-stranded positive-sense RNA genome. Two envelope glycoproteins, E1 and E2, are incorporated in the viral membrane. GBV-C displays a close homology to the genome organization of HCV. The genome consists of 8.9 to 9.4kb and encodes a single ORF predicted to code for a polyprotein of approximately 3000 amino acids[145,157,164,280]. The N-terminal third codes for the structural proteins E1, E2, and p5.6, followed by the nonstructural proteins NS2, NS3, NS4A, NS4B, NS5A, and NS5B[157]. The coding sequence is flanked by untranslated regions (UTR). Hereby, the 5' UTR contains an internal ribosomal entry site (IRES) on which the translation of the viral polyprotein is initiated. Simons *et al.* localized the translational start site to a conserved AUG immediately upstream of the E1 coding region[262]. The relationship between GBV-C and HCV is also reflected in the function of structural and nonstructural proteins. Comparable to HCV, the genome for GBV-C encodes the viral envelope proteins E1 and E2 as well as an ion channel (p5.7). In contrast to HCV, a nucleocapsid of GBV-C has not been found[164]. However, it has been observed that GBV-C infected humans generate antibodies against a putative protein that can be translated from an in-frame upstream AUG suggesting that such a capsid protein is expressed in infected humans[233,313]. There might be a hidden capsid-reading frame in the GBV-C genome. In this regard, it has been noted that a small basic protein is potentially coded in the reading frame of the E2 or in an alternate reading frame of the NS5A protein[148,216]. Alternatively, GBV-C usurps a capsid-like protein from the host cell or a co-infecting virus. Nonstructural GBV-C proteins show the greatest similarity to HCV. The NS2 protein represents an autoprotease. NTP-dependent RNA unwinding helicase and trypsin-like serine protease activity has been demonstrated for the NS3 protein. NS4A serves as a co-factor for the NS3 protease. Although the detailed function is unknown, the NS4B protein may be a replicase component supporting the development of membrane structures, which are associated with the endoplasmatic reticulum (ER). The NS5A protein represents an interferon sensitivity determinant and the NS5B protein codes the viral RNA-dependent RNA polymerase[18,22,137,157].

### 3.2.2. Replication

In contrast to HCV, hepatocytes are not the primary replication site for GBV-C. Rather, GBV-C replicates in the PBMC subsets of CD4 and CD8 positive T lymphocytes as well as CD19 positive B lymphocytes suggesting that GBV-C is a panlymphotropic virus[88,101,155,292]. In addition, it was demonstrated that RNA transcripts from a full-length cDNA clone of GBV-C are infectious in primary CD4 positive T lymphocytes[318]. Although analysis of GBV-C RNA replication is still at an early stage, this process appears to be similar to that of other flaviviruses. Binding and uptake of GBV-C are believed to involve receptor-mediated endocytosis induced by interaction of the E2 protein with one or more cellular receptors. Fusion of the viral envelope with the lipid membrane of the host cell delivers the RNA genome to the cytoplasm, where translation occurs. The IRES within the 5' UTR initiates cap-independent translation of the GBV-C genome. Thereby, the viral proteins are produced as part of a single polyprotein that is co- and post-translational cleaved by cellular and viral proteases. The structural proteins seem to be released by ER-resident cellular signal peptidases[164,262]. E1 and E2 are believed to mature in the ER and to assemble as heterodimers. Cleavage of the nonstructural proteins is mediated by the viral proteases. Whereas the NS2 autoprotease cleaves at the NS2/NS3 junction, the NS3 serine protease mediates cleavages of NS3/NS4, NS4/NS5A, and NS5A/NS5B. Thereby, cleavage of the NS4B/NS5A junction requires expression of the NS4A cofactor[18,157]. Following translation and processing of the viral proteins, it is supposed that viral replication begins with the synthesis of genome-length minus-strand RNA that serves as a template for the synthesis of additional plus-strand RNA[5]. According to HCV, GBV-C replication seems to occur in association with perinuclear membranes and involves the viral polymerase, helicase, and other nonstructural proteins[22,59,77,81,231]. Because of the lack of an efficient cell culture system, events of GBV-C replication like assembly and budding are only poorly understood.

### 3.2.3. Transmission, Prevalence, and Etiopathology

GBV-C can be detected in a relatively high proportion of recipients of blood transfusions, patients on hemodialysis, and intravenous drugs abusers (IVDU). Although parenteral transmission is well documented, other routes of infection, such as vertical and sexual, have also been suggested[7,83,89,91,134,159,163,251,254,268,301]. GBV-C prevalence varies in terms of the geographical origin of the study population as well as of the test system. GBV-C viremia, as defined by the presence of viral RNA in sera or plasma, has been found in 1% to 6% of blood donors in the US and Europe, whereas in Africa up to 18% of the healthy population are positive for GBV-C RNA[66,111,166,290]. Patients with an increased risk of acquiring blood-borne viruses have a higher GBV-C prevalence. In patients, who have a history of chronic hepatitis, multiple blood transfusions or transplantation, prevalence ranged between 10% and 36% [7,52,95,132,164]. In up to 41% of IVDU and HIV positive patients GBV-C virus load could be detected[7,28,57,66,82,111,232,261]. GBV-C infection could persist for more than ten years, but the majority of patients would clear the virus within the first two years after infection accompanied by the development of antibodies directed against the GBV-C E2 protein. Thereby, anti-E2 antibodies are detectable for up to 14 years. Simultaneous presence of GBV-C viremia and anti-E2 antibodies is rarely found suggesting that the number of exposures to GBV-C considerably exceeds the number of active infections detected by RT-PCR. Anti-E2 antibodies has been found in 6% to 18% of blood donors and in up to 68% of persons in high-risk groups[28,82,120,146,262,277,278,281,288]. However, in HIV infected individuals clearance of GBV-C viremia without anti-E2 antibodies could be observed[308]. Although GBV-C was commonly found in patients with chronic hepatitis, hepatocellular carcinoma, or liver cirrhosis (10 to 34%), clinical studies did not indicate a role for GBV-C in liver related diseases[28,121,133,135,160,162,212,279]. However, several epidemiological studies suggest a correlation between GBV-C and genomic destabilization, lymphomagenesis, and B cell lymphoproliferative disorders as well as non-Hodgkin lymphomas[67,151,217], but there are a number of limitations of these studies: using retrospective samples obtained for a different study, small cohorts, controls, and data analysis[267]. Due to the high prevalence of GBV-C in HIV positives patients, GBV-C has been investigated in the context of HIV. Several clinical studies could demonstrate that GBV-C viremia correlates with higher CD4 T cell counts and a slower progression of HIV disease in GBV-C/HIV co-infected patients[120,158,320]. In 2001, two large epidemiological studies were published in parallel by Tillmann *et al.* and Xiang *et al.* demonstrating that GBV-C/HIV co-infected individuals have a higher survival probability than GBV-C negative HIV patients[287,317]. Even though, some studies could not confirm the beneficial effect[24,28,38]. Thereby, the contradictory studies may explained by findings of the Multicenter Acquired Immunodeficiency Syndrome Cohort Study for GBV-C viremia. Williams *et al.* could demonstrate that short-term GBV-C viremia was not associated with prolonged survival among HIV-positive men, but long-term GBV-C viremia was significantly associated with prolonged survival. Moreover, Williams *et al.* could show that the loss of GBV-C RNA within five to six years after HIV seroconversion was associated with the poorest prognosis[308]. Additionally, a Bayesian meta-analysis of 11 prospective survival studies could demonstrate that GBV-C infection early in HIV disease was not associate with increased survival. Exclusively, when GBV-C infection was

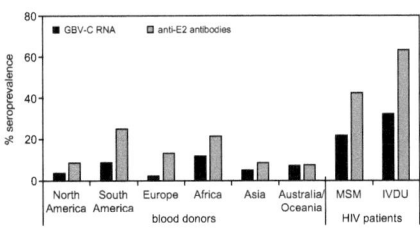

**Figure 3-4: Seroprevalence of GBV-C.** The diagram summarizes the average prevalence of GBV-C RNA indicating GBV-C viremia as well as anti-E2 antibodies indicating a resolved GBV-C infection in volunteer blood donors and HIV-infected patients (men how have sex with men, MSM; intravenous drug users, IVDU) [7,27,28,30,82,111,120,166-168,199,211,277,281,290,308,309].

present later in HIV disease, a significant reduction in the hazard for mortality was observed for those with GBV-C/HIV co-infection[322]. Taken together, the findings of Williams *et al.* and Zhang *et al.* reveal that the timing of GBV-C infection appears to account for the contradictory results of studies on the effect of GBV-C co-infection on survival of HIV-infected people. Interestingly, epidemiological studies suggest that also antibodies elicited by the GBV-C E2 protein mediate a prolonged survival of GBV-C RNA negative, but anti-E2 positive HIV patients[287,308]. However, the exact mechanism of GBV-C/HIV interference remains to be determined. Some studies indicate that GBV-C co-infection leads to changes in the immune homeostasis. Analysis of a prospective cohort study by Nunnari *et al.* reveal an immunological interference of GBV-C with HIV disease progression by maintaining an intact T-helper 1 (Th1) cytokine profile[203]. Changes in the helper T-cell response have a key role in the progression to AIDS. In general, HIV infected patients have a shift in the ratio of the Th1 cytokine level to the Th2 cytokine level in association with HIV disease progression to AIDS. Furthermore, it was published that GBV-C viremia correlates with reduced Fas expression mediating a slower HIV progression of GBV-C/HIV co-infected patients. Fas belongs to the tumor necrosis factor receptor family and plays an important role in immune homeostasis. In the absence of GBV-C, Fas expression on lymphocytes and natural killer cells increases with HIV progression and mediates a higher susceptibility to Fas-mediated apoptosis of HIV infected cells[187]. In addition, it is suggested that HIV replication may be impaired directly or indirectly by GBV-C, possibly through effects on the cell cycle or by stimulation of innate immune mechanisms that inhibit HIV. GBV-C may increase the levels or augment the activity of intracellular HIV inhibitors[224]. GBV-C may also block the entry of HIV into target cells by induction of RANTES and down regulation of CCR5[195,317]. Taken together, a combination of direct antiviral and immune-based effects may be responsible for the beneficial effect of GBV-C on HIV disease progression in patients, who are dually infected with GBV-C and HIV. Understanding of the viral interference might force the success of designing future HIV vaccines and microbicides. While progress has been made in understanding the effect of GBV-C co-infection on HIV progression continued efforts are needed in clinical and basic research to elucidate the mechanism interrelating GBV-C infection and impaired HIV disease progression.

# 4. Aims

Persistent co-infection with the apathogenic GBV-C is associated with higher CD4 T cell counts, lower HIV virus loads, and improved AIDS-free survival leading to a higher survival probability of GBV-C/HIV co-infected individuals[158,171,287,300,317,320]. Surprisingly, not only GBV-C viremia, but also antibodies elicited by the GBV-C E2 protein are associated with increased survival. The question, if GBV-C mediated HIV inhibition is based predominantly on virus-virus interaction or on stimulation of the host's adaptive immune response, remains unanswered so far. The causative relationship between GBV-C infection and HIV suppression was demonstrated earlier by co-infection experiments on primary lymphocytes[129]. Now, the main purpose of this work was to elucidate the mechanism of GBV-C/HIV interference and to identify involved GBV-C proteins. To identify potential viral and cellular determinants affecting the beneficial effect of GBV-C on HIV, several clinical GBV-C isolates and their impact on HIV target cells as well as HIV replication had to be studied. Notably, the GBV-C E2 protein should be investigated, since it was observed that stimulation with recombinant E2 induces CCR5 down regulation[195], which may impair HIV entry. Since HIV positive patients, who have cleared GBV-C infection by the development of anti-E2 antibodies, show also a higher survival probability in comparison to GBV-C negative HIV patients[287,308], a further aim in the course of this study was to analyze the impact of antibodies directed against the GBV-C E2 protein on HIV infectivity.

14

# 5. Results

## 5.1. A Cell Culture System for GB Virus C

GBV-C was classified to be a member of the *Flaviviridae* familiy and is closely related to HCV. As it is described for HCV, also for GBV-C there is currently no efficient cell culture system available that enables investigation of the GBV-C replication process. GBV-C is an apathogentic virus and since epidemiological studies could demonstrate that GBV-C interferes with HIV, it is important to investigate this phenomenon under standardized conditions in cell culture experiments. Therefore, a robust infection system should be developed that provides prolonged cultivation of clinical GBV-C isolates as well as HIV co-infection experiments to study GBV-C/HIV interference. For this purpose, a real-time RT-PCR was developed to quantify GBV-C RNA and to monitor GBV-C replication.

### 5.1.1. A Real-Time RT-PCR to detect GB Virus C RNA

The GBV-C genome is formed by a single, plus-strand RNA molecule that is incorporated in the viral particle. Post infection of susceptible cells, the GBV-C genome is liberated into the cytoplasm, where it is translated into a polyprotein that is processed by cellular and viral proteases. During the replication process, the viral replicase synthesizes also a few copies of minus-strand RNA that serve as templates for the production of excess amounts of viral RNA genomes. To quantify GBV-C RNA in serum, cell culture supernatants, and infected host cells, a real-time RT-PCR was established. Based on sequence alignments, conserved genome regions were identified and a set of oligonucleotide primers located in the 5' UTR were designed and used to produce a GBV-C specific RNA standard. A 93bp DNA fragment that presents the nucleotides 96-188 of the GBV-C clone AF121950, was amplified and cloned into the plasmid pCR2.1-TOPO® to generate the plasmids pCR2.1_Iowa[96-188] and pCR2.1_Iowa[188-96reverse]. To ensure generation of uniform RNA molecules of the same length, the fragment containing the GBV-C insert and the T7 promoter was amplified using the M13 primer set. Transcription by the MEGAscript® T7 kit produced plus- or minus-strand RNA. To remove remaining template DNA, different RNA purification methods were tested. In addition to an initial DNaseI treatment step (DNA-*free*, Applied Biosystems, Darmstadt) as well as removal of divalent cations, remaining DNA/RNA heteroduplexes were purified by a second purification round by phenol/chloroforme extraction, DNA-*free*,

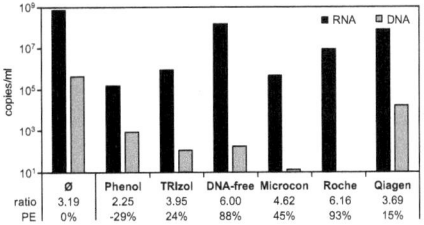

Figure 5-1: Comparison of different RNA purification methods. A 93 nucleotide fragment of the 5' UTR of the GBV-C clone AF121950 was amplified and cloned into the pCR2.1 vector. Transcription by the T7 polymerase produced RNA molecules that were used to generate samples of predefined GBV-C RNA copies per reaction and thereby to establish a GBV-C RNA standard. To remove remaining template DNA, various purification methods were tested. Whereas the amount of RNA/DNA (black columns) was quantified by real-time RT-PCR, DNA molecules (grey columns) were quantified by real-time PCR. RNA/DNA and DNA concentration of the initial sample (Ø) were determined. The ratio of RNA/DNA to DNA as well as the purification efficiency (PE) calculated by the quotient of $\log_{10}(\text{ratio}_{\text{method}})$ and $\log_{10}(\text{ratio}_{\text{initial}})$-1, are shown.

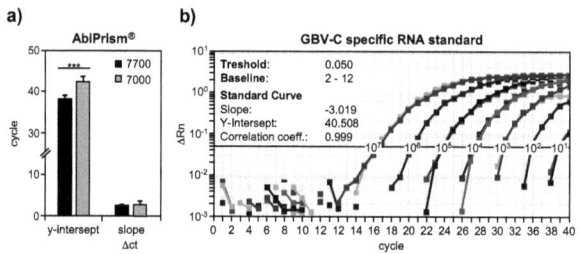

Figure 5-2: Detection of GBV-C RNA using the AbiPrism® 7700 and 7000. To investigate the efficiency and sensitivity of the generated GBV-C RNA standard and the respective real-time RT-PCR, serial dilutions of $10^7$ to $10^1$ genome equivalents per reaction without detectable amounts of DNA were amplified by the SuperScript® III Platinum One-Step qRT-PCR System and the detection systems AbiPrism® 7700 and 7000 (Applied Biosystems, Darmstadt). **a)** Comparison of the detection sensitivity and amplification efficiency of the AbiPrism® 7700 and 7000. Columns represent the average y-intercept (sensitivity) and slope (efficiency) of at least 20 independent real-time RT-PCR. Both devices displayed comparable slopes (3.15 vs. 3.40) corresponding to an efficiency of 108% vs. 97% as well as a similar sensitivity (y-intercept: 35.23 vs. 40.51). **b)** The line chart illustrates the amplification of the generated GBV-C specific RNA standard by a typical real-time RT-PCR on the AbiPrism® 7000 system using the reaction kit described above. A single experiment performed in duplicates is shown.

Microcon-100 (Millipore, Schwalbach) or column-based purification kits (High Pure RNA Isolation System, Roche Diagnostics, Mannheim; QIAamp Viral RNA Mini Kit, Qiagen, Hilden). To investigate the efficiency of the different purification methods, the ratio of RNA to contaminating DNA before and after the additional purification step, was determined by real-time PCR with and without reverse transcription. After the initial purification step, the sample contained $7.0 \times 10^8$ RNA and $4.5 \times 10^5$ DNA copies per milliliter corresponding to a ratio of 3.19. In comparison, the RNA to DNA ratio of each sample was calculated and efficiency of the respective purification method was determined. Hereby, column-based purification methods (DNA-*free*, Microcon-100) provided an increased RNA recovery rate, a better elimination of contaminating DNA, and thereby a higher purification efficiency than the phenol-dependent purification methods (phenol/chloroform, TRIzol). The RNA purification kit from Roche gave the best results. Whereas just one log of the initial RNA was lost, the DNA contamination of $4.5 \times 10^5$ copies per reaction could be removed completely (Figure 5-1). The concentration of purified RNA was determined by the absorption of light at 260nm and 280nm and used to calculate the RNA molecule number via the specific molecular weigth of the expected RNA fragment. Serial dilutions ranging from $1 \times 10^7$ to $1 \times 10^0$ genome equivalents per reaction were assayed together with negative control reactions using the AbiPrism® 7700 and 7700 (Applied Biosystems, Darmstadt) as well as the SuperScript® III Platinum One-Step Quantitative RT-PCR and the Platinum Quantitative RT-PCR ThermoScript® One-Step kit (Invitrogen, Groningen). Standard curves were generated by plotting the $\Delta$ct values against the decadic logarithm of the initial copy number (Figure 5-2). PCR amplification efficiency (E) was calculated by the average $\Delta$ct value (slope) and the equation: $E = 10^{(-1/\text{slope})} - 1$. Slopes between -3.1 and -3.6 giving efficiencies between 90% and 110%, are typically acceptable, which means that the amplicon quantity doubles with every cycle. Independent of the used assay kit both AbiPrism® detection systems provided an overall sensitivity of approximatly $5 \times 10^2$ molecules per milliliter. The efficiency ranged between 108% (AbiPrism® 7700, slope 3.15) and 97% (AbiPrism® 7000, slope 3.40). For further real-time RT-PCR the AbiPrim® 7000 was used.

## 5.1.2. Limited Replication of GB Virus C in Human B and T Cell Lines

The clinical impact of GBV-C on HIV progression rapidly led to the delineation of the genomic organization and the structural as well as biochemical characterization of several GBV-C proteins. However, studies of the viral life cycle and elucidation of the detailed mechanism of GBV-C/HIV interference have been hampered by the lack of a robust and reliable cell culture system. The liver is not the primary replication site for GBV-C[155] and several studies demonstrate that GBV-C replicates predominantly in lymphocytes[88,101,318]. Therefore, different human B and T cell lines were analyzed in terms of GBV-C susceptibility. $5 \times 10^5$ Bjab, Raji, P3HR-1, CEMx174, Jurkat, or PM1 cells were incubated over night in a total volume of 500µl RPMI$_{complete}$ with 10µl serum of the GBV-C donor 10750 corresponding to $2 \times 10^6$ GBV-C genome equivalents. Cells were washed twice in 50ml PBS, resuspended in RPMI$_{complete}$, adjusted to $1 \times 10^5$ cells per milliliter, and cultivated under standard growth conditions. At different time points, cells and cell-free supernatants were harvested and stored at -80°C until viral RNA was extracted and quantified by real-time RT-PCR. Although GBV-C was detectable in all cell lines for a time period of 28 days, GBV-C RNA concentration in cell lysates and cell culture supernatants was very low and reached at most $4.9 \times 10^4$ GBV-C genome equivalents per milliliter. Whereas GBV-C RNA could be detected in Raji, P3HR-1, and Jurkat cells just during the first 7 to 17 days post infection, prolonged propagation of GBV-C for at least four weeks was observed in Bjab, CEMx174, and PM1 cells (Figure 5-3). The data suggest that established B and T cell lines provide just an inefficient cultivation of GBV-C and were not suitable to establish a robust cell culture system for GBV-C.

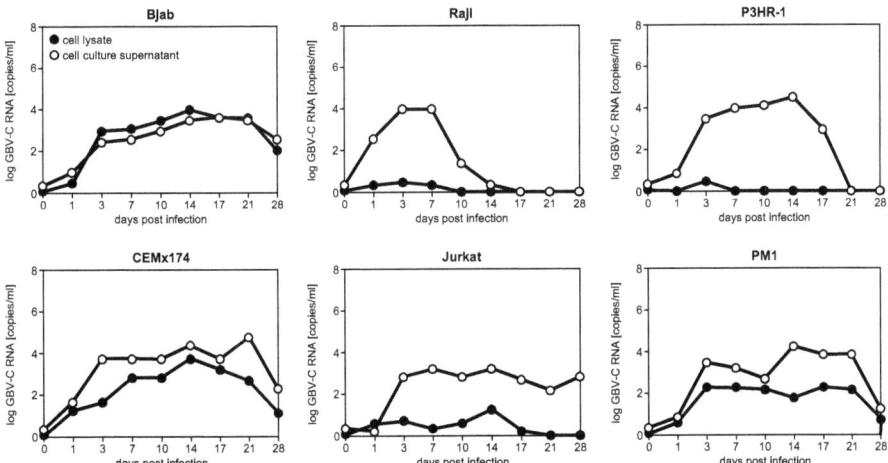

**Figure 5-3: Replication of GBV-C on human B and T cell lines.** $5 \times 10^5$ Bjab, Raji, and P3HR-1 cells (B cell lines) as well as $5 \times 10^5$ CEMx174, Jurkat, and PM1 cells (T cell lines) were infected over night with 100µl of the GBV-C positive serum 10750 corresponding to $2 \times 10^6$ GBV-C genome equivalents in total volume of 500µl RPMI$_{complete}$. Cells were washed, maintained in RPMI$_{complete}$, and cultivated under standard growth conditions for at least four weeks. At different time points, cells and cell-free supernatants were collected and GBV-C virus load was quantified by real-time RT-PCR.

### 5.1.3. Increased Replication of GB Virus C in Human Lymphocytes

Since infection and productive virus replication can depend on the interplay between different cell types and/or on host cell factors that are sometimes expressed only in differentiated primary cells, PBMC from healthy volunteers were isolated by Ficoll-Hypaque density centrifugation. CD4 and CD19 positive lymphocytes were enriched by magnetic cell separation. Cells were cultivated for at least two days under standard growth conditions in the presence of 10U/ml IL-2 and 10µg/ml PHA. To investigate the GBV-C susceptibility of PBMC, CD4, and CD19 cells, $5 \times 10^6$ cells were resuspended in 400µl RPMI$_{complete}$ and inoculated with 100µl serum of the GBV-C donor 10750 corresponding to $2 \times 10^7$ GBV-C genome equivalents and ongoing GBV-C replication was monitored by real-time RT-PCR. Additionally, two days post GBV-C infection, $5 \times 10^4$ cells were harvested, washed, and stained with anti-E2 antibodies directed against the GBV-C envelope protein E2 (Figure 5-4). Comparable to previously tested cell lines, primary lymphocytes enabled just a moderate GBV-C replication. However, GBV-C RNA could be detected in cell lysates and cell culture supernatants for at least four weeks suggesting that primary cells are more susceptible for GBV-C than human cell lines. Indeed, immunofluorescence of infected lymphocytes proved the expression of the E2 protein and indicated GBV-C replication. Besides lymphocytes from adult volunteers, also cord blood lymphocytes (CBL) that are less differentiated than PBMC, but still express a wide spectrum of cellular receptors, were investigated. Within six hours post delivery, cord blood donations without supplements were processed. $5 \times 10^6$ CBL of three donors were infected with GBV-C positive sera, normalized to $2 \times 10^7$ GBV-C genome equivalents. Infection was performed for four hours in 1ml RPMI$_{complete}$. Cells were washed, maintained in 2ml RPMI$_{complete}$ supplemented with 10U/ml IL-2, and cultivated under standard growth conditions.

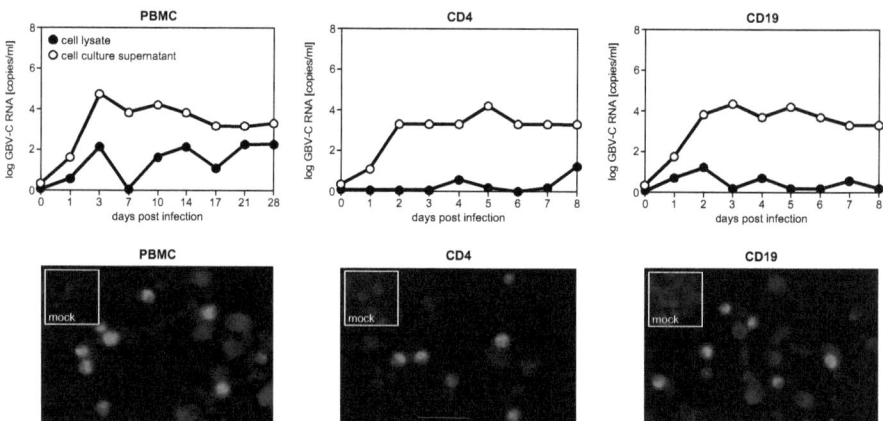

**Figure 5-4: Replication of GBV-C on PBMC.** PBMC were isolated by Ficoll-Hypaque density centrifugation and CD4 and CD19 positive cells were enriched by magnetic beads separation and cultivated for at least two days in RPMI$_{complete}$ (10U/ml IL-2, 10µg/ml PHA). For GBV-C infection, $5 \times 10^6$ cells were harvested, washed, and infected over night with 100µl of the GBV-C positive serum 10750 corresponding to $2 \times 10^6$ GBV-C genome equivalents in total volume of 500µl RPMI$_{complete}$. At the next day, the cells were washed, resuspended in growth medium, and cultivated for at least eight days. At different time points, cells and cell-free supernatants were collected and GBV-C virus load was quantified by real-time RT-PCR. Additional, at day 2 post GBV-C infection $5 \times 10^5$ cells were collected and stained for expression of the GBV-C E2 protein (mouse anti-E2, goat anti-mouse FITC, green) in relation to mock infected cells.

In addition, selected viruses were passaged to prove active replication. 1ml cell-free supernatant was transferred to fresh CBL, incubated overnight, and GBV-C virus load was quantified at different time points. GBV-C RNA concentration in the supernatants of infected CBL corresponds in average to $10^6$ molecules per milliliter, even though, depending of the GBV-C isolates, up to $10^8$ copies per milliliter could be measured as well (Figure 5-5). In general, GBV-C RNA concentration of infected CBL was up to two log higher than for the investigated B and T cell lines. Furthermore, cell-free supernatants of GBV-C infected CBL were sufficient to infect fresh CBL. Even though, the virus load in the second and third passage was lower than for the primary GBV-C infection. Although slight differences in the replication ability of different GBV-C isolates could be observed, CBL represent an efficient system to study GBV-C replication.

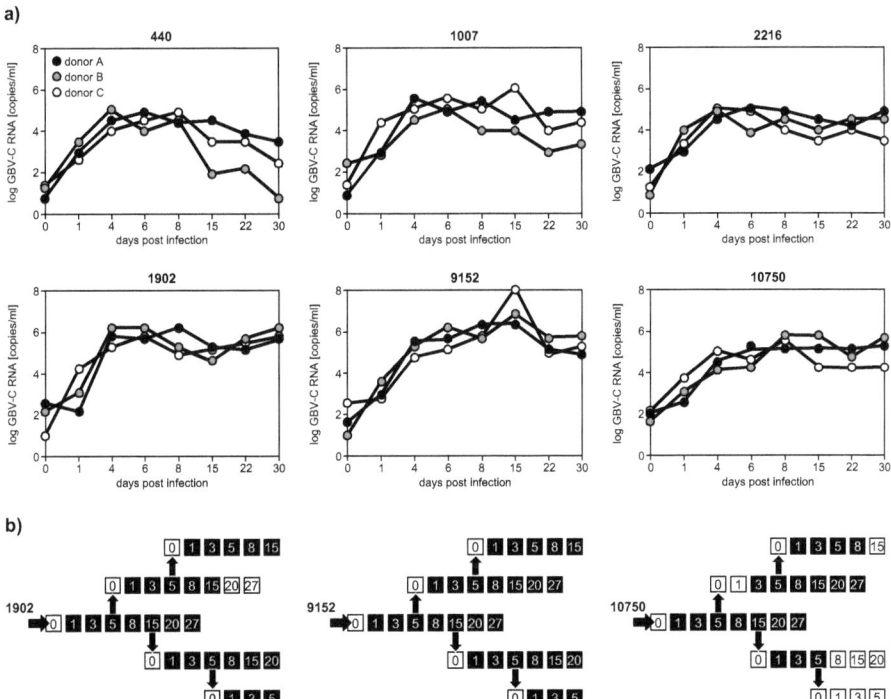

**Figure 5-5: Replication of GBV-C on CBL.** CBL were isolated by Ficoll-Hypaque density centrifugation and infected with GBV-C RNA positive sera of several donors. The infectious dose was normalized to GBV-C genome equivalents per milliliter. Four hours post infection, cells were washes, and resuspended in RPMI$_{complete}$ (10U/ml IL-2, 10µg/ml PHA). Supernatants were harvested at different time points and GBV-C virus load was quantified by real-time RT-PCR. **a)** Line charts represent the replication capacity of six GBV-C isolates (440, 1007, 2216, 1902, 9152, 10750) on CBL derived from three different donors. **b)** CBL were infected with three GBV-C isolates (1902, 9152, 10750). At day 5 and day 15, cell-free supernatants were harvested and used to infect fresh CBL (black arrows). Each line of squares represents an individual GBV-C infection or GBV-C passage. Numbers within the squares indicate the days post infections. Whereas black squares represent detectable amounts of GBV-C RNA, white squares indicate GBV-C RNA negative samples. A single experiment performed in duplicates with two different blood donors is shown.

## 5.2. Variability of Clinical GB Virus C Isolates

Epidemiological studies suggest a beneficial effect for GBV-C/HIV co-infected individuals leading to a delayed progression of HIV disease and an increased probability to survive. To investigate the clinical relevance of GBV-C infection on HIV disease progression, cell culture experiments were necessary.

### 5.2.1. A GB Virus C Sera Bank

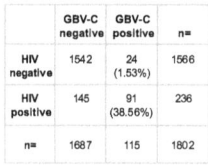
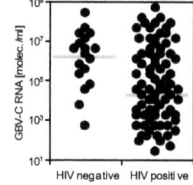

**Figure 5-6: Correlation of GBV-C virus load and HIV status.** Sera of 1802 volunteers were screened for GBV-C and HIV RNA. GBV-C virus load was quantified by real-time RT-PCR (left) and grouped according to the HIV status of the blood donor. Each dot represents a single donor, grey bars indicate the geometric mean of the distinct groups (right).

In cooperation with Prof. Hans L. Tillmann (University of Leipzig) a GBV-C sera bank was established and used to investigate the impact of GBV-C on HIV replication. Serum samples of 1566 blood donors of the Leipzig and Erlangen area as well as of 236 HIV patients were collected. Viral RNA was isolated and samples were screened for GBV-C viremia (Figure 5-6). GBV-C RNA could be detected in 24 HIV negative (1.5%) and 91 HIV positive samples (38.6%). The average GBV-C virus load in HIV negative donors was higher than in HIV positive donors ($3.0 \times 10^6$ vs. $5.4 \times 10^4$ genome equivalents per milliliter), but the difference was not significant (p=0.5, Student's t-Test). GBV-C virus load varied between $5 \times 10^2$ and $8 \times 10^8$ GBV-C genome equivalents per milliliter (Figure 5-6). For further experiments, multiple aliquots corresponding to $4.0 \times 10^6$ genome equivalents or 500µl were stored at -80°C.

### 5.2.2. Differences in the Replication Capacity of Clinical GB Virus C Isolates

Since GBV-C virus load displays a great variability, it should be investigated, if observed differences are caused by the replication capacity of the respective GBV-C isolate. Multiple blood samples of GBV-C viremic volunteers were collected within a period of six to twelve months and average GBV-C virus load in blood plasma (*in vivo*) was calculated as the arithmetic mean of at least three single quantifications. Additionally, PBMC of GBV-C viremic blood donors were isolated and cultivated for three to four weeks. At different time points, supernatants were collected and GBV-C RNA was quantified. The GBV-C virus load in cell culture supernatants of naturally infected PBMC (*ex vivo*) was then calculated from at least seven individual measurements. GBV-C *ex vivo* replication capacity ranged from nearly undetectable to $10^7$ GBV-C RNA copies per milliliter. Hereby, the average virus load in the supernatants of isolated PBMC of GBV-C viremic donors was always lower than the average GBV-C RNA concentration in serum or plasma of the respective donor. A direct correlation between the GBV-C virus load *ex vivo* and *in vivo* could not be observed (Figure 5-7). Additionally, the average difference between *ex vivo* and *in vivo* was calculated in relation to the HIV status of the blood donor (HIV positive: D0223, 440, 2216, 10750; HIV negative: D0306, D1007, D1108, D1902, D1920) and was slightly higher in HIV positive than in HIV negative GBV-C donors (3.1 log vs. 2.7 log).

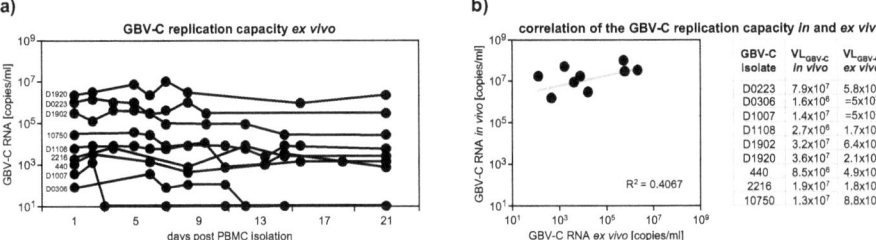

**Figure 5-7: Variability of the replication capacity of clinical GBV-C isolates.** PBMC of nine blood donors with active GBV-C viremia (D0223, D0306, D1007, D1108, D1902, D1920, 440, 2216, 10750) were isolated and cultivated in RPMI$_{complete}$ (10U/ml IL-2, 10µg/ml PHA) for up to three weeks. At different time points, cell culture supernatants were collected and GBV-C virus load was quantified. **a)** Each line chart illustrates the replication capacity of a single GBV-C isolate on natural infected PBMC (*ex vivo*). **b)** Within a period of three weeks, GBV-C virus load in cell culture supernatant of natural infected PBMC (*ex vivo*) was determined. Even though, the average GBV-C virus load in serum or plasma of the respective GBV-C donor (*in vivo*) of at least three independent samples was quantified and compared with the average *ex vivo* GBV-C virus load.

### 5.2.3. Sequence Divergence of Clinical GB Virus C Isolates

GBV-C is an ancient virus and it has been shown to exist as a group of six closely related genotypes that showed consistent geographical clustering. Although clinical GBV-C isolates display a great variation of their replication capacity, observed differences could neither be explained by the virus load in blood plasma of the respective blood donor nor by HIV co-infection. To investigate, if the replication variability of clinical GBV-C isolates could be explained by their genotype, viral RNA was isolated, reverse transcribed, amplified, and sequenced according to the method described by Sanger *et al.*[243,244]. A 1457nt comprising fragment of the GBV-C E2 protein corresponding to nt987-2447 of the GBV-C isolate AF121950, were aligned with reference strains of the six known GBV-C genotypes. The GBV-C isolates 2216, 4080, 9152, D1007, D1506, D1902 were classified to be genotype 2a, whereas the isolate 10750 was classified as genotype 5. Since genotype 2a and 5 isolates display comparable virus loads in humans ($10^6$ to $10^7$ GBV-C genome equivalents per milliliter) and furthermore, the GBV-C isolate 10750 is characterized by a low virus load on isolated, naturally infected PBMC ($8.8 \times 10^3$ GBV-C genome equivalents per milliliter), but high a hight GBV-C virus load in blood plasma ($1.3 \times 10^7$ GBV-C genome equivalents per milliliter), it seems unusual that the replication capacity of GBV-C depends on a certain genotype.

The E2 protein of HCV has a hypervariable region (HVR) that is thought to be a neutralizing epitope facilitating HCV persistence by selection of escape variants from the HVR quasispecies pool[205,305]. It is suggested that the GBV-C E2 protein contains also replaceable amino acids, which might be part of an antigenic region[280]. To investigate, if GBV-C replication variablity is related to distinct mutations within the E2 protein, E2 amino acid sequences were deduced and aligned. Thereby, GBV-C isolates were grouped according their *ex vivo* virus load on isolated, naturally infected PBMC of the respective GBV-C viremic blood donor. A HVR could not be identified. However, clinical GBV-C isolates have accumulated different mutations leading to amino acid substitutions that are spread over the entire E2 sequence. Interestingly, two amino acids were mutated exclusively in the E2 protein of GBV-C isolates that are characterized by a

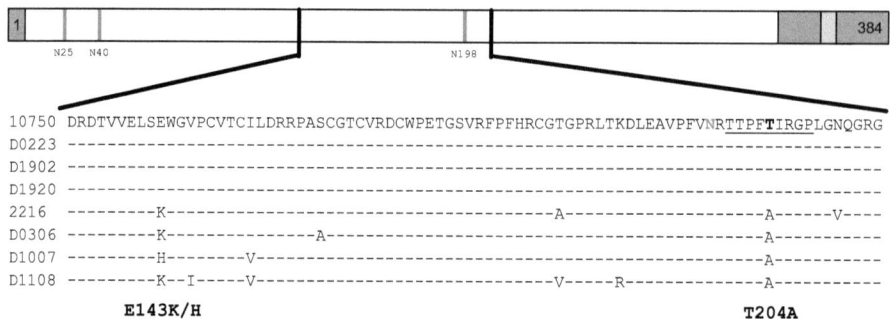

**Figure 5-8: Mutations in the amino acid sequence of the envelope protein E2 of clinical GBV-C isolates.** The figure illustrates the GBV-C E2 protein with the cytoplasma and transmembrane domains (grey) as well as the three N-linked glycosylation sites (green bars). Numbers indicate the respective amino acid. E2 amino acid sequences, deduced from the nucleotide sequences of uncloned GBV-C isolates, were aligned and grouped according their GBV-C virus load *ex vivo* (=1.7x10⁴ GBV-C genome equivalents per milliliter: 2216, D0306, D1007, D1108 and =5.8x10⁵ GBV-C genome equivalents per milliliter: 10750, D0223, D1902, D1920). A fragment corresponding to amino acid 133-215 is shown and displays the majority of observed amino acid substitutions.

virus load *ex vivo* lower than 1x10$^5$ GBV-C genome equivalents per milliliter (Figure 5-8). The glutamate at position 143 was replaced either by lysine or histidine (E143K/H). The threonine at position 200 was substituted by alanine (T204A). To locate the substituted amino acids and to determine their relevance for protein folding and protein-protein interactions, 3D models of mutated E2 proteins were calculated, using the I-TASSER server[323]. Sequence pattern for post-transcriptional modifications as well as B cell epitopes were identified by ppsearch (www.ebi.ac.uk), DiscoTop, Bepipred, and Seppa, respectively[117,154,272]. E143 is highly exposed on the E2 surface and substitution by lysine or histidine leads to a charge shift from negative to positive. T204 is located hidden in a protein cavern and part of a predicted linear B cell epitope as well as of a phosphate kinase c phosphorylation site that is deleted by the T204A mutation.

## 5.3. Interference of GB Virus C with Human Immunodeficiency Virus

Immunosuppression facilitates different fungal, bacterial, and viral co-infections in patients suffering from HIV. Due to similar transmission routes, GBV-C infection was investigated in the context of HIV. Many studies confirm an increased prevalence of GBV-C viremia in HIV infected patients. However, in contrast to the expectations, GBV-C does not exacerbate the course of HIV. Longitudinal studies demonstrate that GBV-C leads to a slower progression to AIDS. Even though, the underlying mechanism is still unknown.

### 5.3.1. Classification of Clinical GB Virus C Isolates as HIV-Inhibitory and HIV-Non-Inhibitory

In earlier work I could demonstrate that co-infection of PBMC with GBV-C and HIV leads to significant suppression of HIV replication, which was independent of the co-receptor tropism and the origin of the HIV isolate[129]. The data were confirmed by HIV infection experiments on GBV-C RNA transfected PBMC. Transfection of plus-strand full length RNA hampered the replication of HIV in relation to cells that were transfected by non-coding minus-strand full length RNA[131].

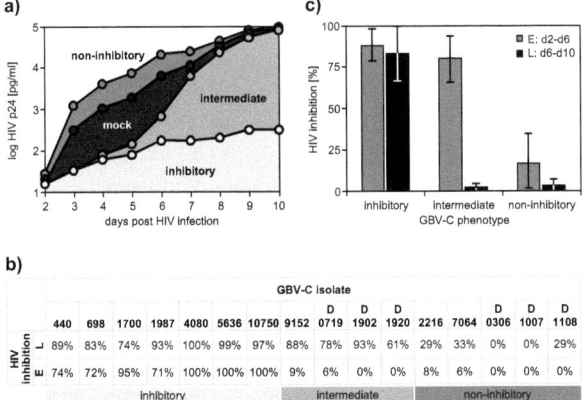

Figure 5-9: Clinical GBV-C isolates differ in their HIV-inhibitory phenotype. PBMC were infected with several clinical GBV-C isolates, normalized by GBV-C genome equivalents, washed, and cultivated for at least two days. HIV infection using different primary HIV isolates were performed and HIV replication was monitored by p24 antigen concentration in the supernatants. a) Three prototypes of HIV replication curves on GBV-C infected PBMC could be observed and were used to classify GBV-C isolates according their HIV-inhibitory phenotype as HIV-inhibitory, HIV-non-inhibitory, and intermediate. Line charts illustrate the impact on HIV replication by different phenotypes. For better differentiation and comparability of the different prototypes of GBV-C mediated HIV inhibition the respective areas under curve were colored. b) Area under curve for early (E, d02-d06) and late (L, d06-d10) phase of HIV infection was determined for each GBV-C isolate and used to calculate HIV inhibition in relation to mock. The table summarizes the short- (E) and long-term (L) HIV-inhibitory capacity of 16 GBV-C isolates. c) GBV-C isolates were grouped according their HIV-inhibitory phenotype and average inhibition was calculated.

To investigate the impact of several clinical GBV-C isolates on HIV replication, co-infection experiments were performed. Interestingly, GBV-C isolates differed in their ability to inhibit HIV replication and three distinct HIV-inhibitory phenotypes could be identified. Whereas the majority of GBV-C isolates displayed a strong inhibition of HIV and were classified as HIV-inhibitory isolates, some GBV-C isolates did not influence the HIV replication at all and were classified as HIV-non-inhibitory. A minority of GBV-C isolates displayed an intermediate phenotype and suppressed HIV only within the first days of HIV co-infection (Figure 5-9).

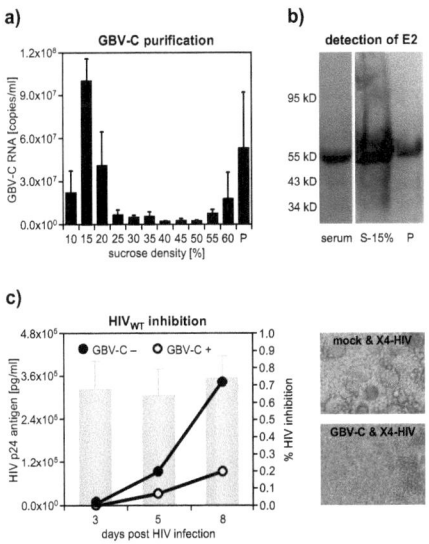

Figure 5-10: Inhibition of $HIV_{WT}$ by purified GBV-C virions. a) Sera of GBV-C RNA positives were purified by sucrose density centrifugation (200000g, 3.5h, 4°C). Fractions were collected and GBV-C viral load was determined by real-time RT-PCR. b) Serum as well as the 15% sucrose fraction (S-15%) and the centrifugation pellet (P) that displayed the highest GBV-C RNA titers were centrifuged at 200000g for 1 hour at 4°C. Pellets were mixed with an equal volume of reducing sample buffer and boiled for 10 minutes before samples were subjected to a 5%/10% discontinuous sodium dodecyl sulfate (SDS) polyacrylamide gel. The polyacrylamide gel was processed for Western blotting and stained for the GBV-C envelope protein E2 (~55kD) using a monoclonal anti-E2 antibody. c) CEMx174 cells were inoculated with equal volumes of S-15% derived either by centrifugation of GBV-C RNA positive serum or by centrifugation of mock sera (GBV-C RNA negative) two days prior infection with the CXCR4-tropic isolate 92UG024 was performed. HIV replication was analyzed by p24 (line charts) and HIV inhibition was calculated in relation to mock (columns). Furthermore, HIV suppression was monitored by syncytia formation on GBV-C/HIV co-infected or mock infected CEMx174 cells (pictures, right).

To exclude unspecific effects by human serum proteins, GBV-C virions were purified by discontinuous sucrose density gradient centrifugation. Sera of GBV-C RNA positive and negative blood donors were overlaid on a sucrose density gradient composed of 60%, 50%, 40%, 30%, 20%, and 10% (wt/vol) sucrose solutions and centrifuged at 200000g for 3.5 hours at 4°C in a Beckman Coulter SW41Ti rotor. Fractions were aspirated from the top of the gradient. The RNA titer of each fraction was quantified by real-time RT-PCR. The highest GBV-C concentrations could be determined in the fraction containing 15% sucrose (S-15%) as well as in the pellet (P). SDS-Page and western blot analysis using anti-E2 antibodies proved the presence of viral particles. To exclude assay variation and artificial HIV inhibition due to the genetic diversity of different PBMC donors, co-infection experiments were repeated using purified GBV-C virions and the human T cell line CEMx174. Therefore, CEMx174 cells were inoculated with comparable volumes of fraction S-15% derived from GBV-C RNA negative serum or fraction S-15% derived from serum of an HIV-inhibitory GBV-C isolate prior HIV infection was performed. Comparable to previous co-infection experiments using GBV-C positive sera, purified GBV-C particles inhibited HIV as well. The inhibitory effect was also visible by a delay in the formation of HIV-induced syncytia (Figure 5-10). Single round of infection assays using HIV pseudoparticles (HIV$_{PP}$) bearing homologous HIV$_{gp120}$ or heterologous VSV$_G$ envelopes, were performed to investigate the HIV-inhibitory capacity of clinical GBV-C isolates in more detail. The use of replication deficient HIV$_{PP}$ offers a more sensitive infection assay than HIV wildtype (HIV$_{WT}$) infections, since this assay monitors only one replication cycle and prevents masking of an HIV-inhibitory effect by several replication rounds. Moreover, the system allows modification of the entry mechanism of HIV$_{PP}$. HIV$_{PP}$ enveloped with HIV$_{gp120}$ bind to CD4 and CCR5 or CXCR4, respectively and enable infection by receptor mediated fusion[48,71,80]. VSV$_G$ pseudoparticles elude HIV receptor binding mechanisms and enter target cells by endocytosis[274]. HIV$_{PP}$ were produced by transfection of 293T cells with pNL4-3lucR-E- and an envelope expression vector without HIV packaging signal. pNL4-3lucR-E- codes for the HIV *gag-pol* gene of the HIV isolate NL4-3 and a firefly luciferase gene that was inserted into the *nef* gene. Furthermore, it contains two frameshifts that render this clone env- and vpr-[58,118]. Two days post transfection, supernatants were harvested and used to infect GBV-C stimulated cells. Replication capacity of HIV$_{PP}$ was quantified three days later by the luciferase activity in the cell lysates. Comparable to HIV$_{WT}$, HIV$_{PP}$ were inhibited by GBV-C. Again, the same HIV-inhibitory and non-inhibitory phenotypes were observed. Whereas GBV-C isolates, classified as HIV-inhibitory, suppressed HIV$_{gp120}$ and VSV$_G$ enveloped HIV$_{PP}$, HIV-non-inhibitory GBV-C isolates did not. Interstingly, intermediate GBV-C isolates

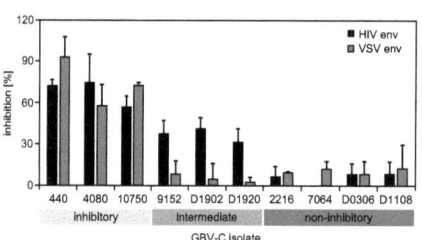

Figure 5-11: Inhibition of HIV$_{PP}$ by clinical GBV-C isolates. CEMx174 cells were infected with different GBV-C isolates, washed, maintained in growth medium and cultivated for two days prior infection with HIV$_{PP}$ was performed. HIV$_{PP}$ were enveloped either with the gp120 protein of NL4-3 or with the glycoprotein G of VSV. Three days later, cells were lysed and luciferase activity was measured. Inhibition was calculated in relation to mock. Average inhibition of at least five experiments performed in triplicates is shown.

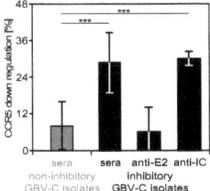

Figure 5-12: Down regulation of CCR5 surface expression by HIV-inhibitory GBV-C isolates. PBMC of healthy volunteers were infected with GBV-C positive sera in relation to GBV-C negative (mock) sera. CCR5 expression was determined by FACS 24, 48, 72, 96, 120, and 168 hours post infection. Six GBV-C isolates were investigated in at least three independent experiments. Average down regulation was calculated for each GBV-C isolate in relation to mock and used to calculate the average reduction of CCR5 expression of the respective HIV-inhibitory phenotype (non-inhibitory or inhibitory). To prove the specificity of the observed effect, serum of a HIV-inhibitory GBV-C isolate was preincubated either with anti-E2 or isotype control (IC) antibodies.

inhibited exclusively $HIV_{gp120}$ enveloped $HIV_{PP}$. The data corroborate the existence of different HIV-inhibitory phenotypes and suggest that GBV-C impairs HIV by an $HIV_{gp120}$-dependent mechanism. Whereas potent HIV-inhibitory GBV-C isolates affect HIV entry and post-entry replication steps, weak HIV-inhibitory GBV-C isolates with intermediate phenotype impair exclusively HIV entry (Figure 5-11). Since HIV entry is affected by expression of CD4, CCR5, and CXCR4, PBMC were infected with HIV-inhibitory and HIV-non-inhibitory GBV-C isolates and receptor expression was investigated by flow cytometry using monoclonal phycoerythrin (PE) conjugated murine anti-CD4, anti-CCR5 or anti-CXCR4 antibodies (Becton Dickinson, Heidelberg). Whereas extracellular expression of CD4 and CXCR4 was not affected, HIV-inhibitory GBV-C isolates induced a significant down regulation of CCR5. Specificity could be proved by preincubation of serum derived from an HIV-inhibitory GBV-C isolate with anti-E2 antibodies that abolished the effect (Figure 5-12). Expression of the HIV co-recptors CCR5 and CXCR4 is affected by the beta-chemokines RANTES, MIP-1alpha, and MIP-1beta as well as by the alpha-chemokine SDF-1, respectively[10,11,54]. Chemokine induction by GBV-C positive sera was analyzed by ELISA. Exclusively HIV-inhibitory GBV-C isolates stimulated the secretion of beta-chemokines, whereas no induction of SDF-1 could be observed. Even though, chemokine induction by HIV-inhibitory GBV-C isolates was specifically blocked by preincubation of the GBV-C inoculum with anti-E2 antibodies (Figure 5-13). Although induction of beta-chemokines might explain reduced CCR5 expression and inhibition of CCR5-tropic HIV, observed inhibition of CXCR4-tropic $HIV_{WT}$ as well as $VSV_G$ enveloped $HIV_{PP}$ could not be explained by GBV-C mediated chemokine secretion.

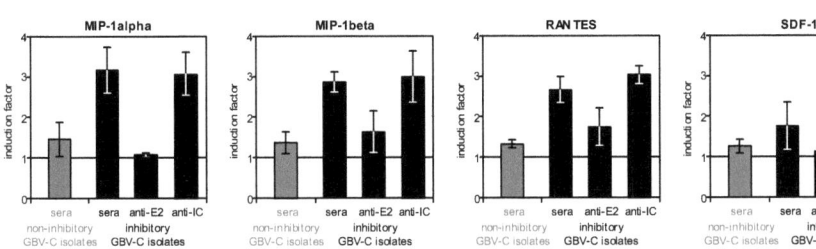

Figure 5-13: Chemokine induction by HIV-inhibitory GBV-C isolates. PBMC of healthy volunteers were infected with GBV-C positive and GBV-C negative (mock) sera. Cell culture supernatants were collected 4, 24, 48, 72, 96, 120, 144, and 168 hours post infection and concentrations of MIP-1alpha, MIP-1beta, RANTES, and SDF-1 were determined by ELISA. Six GBV-C isolates were investigated in at least three independent experiments. Average induction factors were calculated for each GBV-C isolate in relation to mock and used to calculate the average chemokine induction depending of the HIV-inhibitory phenotype (non-inhibitory or inhibitory). Induction factors higher than one indicate stimulation of chemokine secretion. To prove the specificity of the observed effect, serum of a HIV-inhibitory GBV-C isolate was preincubated with anti-E2 or with isotype control (IC) antibodies.

## 5.3.2. HIV Impairment by Expression of GB Virus C Gene Cassettes in a Rhadinovirus Vector System

To narrow down HIV-inhibitory GBV-C proteins, a *Herpesvirus saimiri* (HVS) strain C488 based vector system, developed by the group of Prof. A. Ensser and Prof. Fleckenstein (University Hospital Erlangen), was used to generate human T cell lines that stable express overlapping GBV-C gene cassettes. $HVS_{C488}$ represents the prototyp of the gamma-2-herpesviruses and is able to persist in squirrel monkeys (*Saimiri sciureus*) without any apparent disease. Even though, virtually all T lymphocytes become infected. Certain subgroup C virus strains are capable to transform human T lymphocytes. Thereby, transformed T cells harbor multiple copies of the HVS genome in form of stable, non-integrated episomes, do not produce HVS particles, and maintain the antigen specificity and many other functions of their parental T cell clone[84]. Overlapping GBV-C gene cassettes were cloned into pRSETB_$P_{CMV}$ to generate CMV promoter driven GBV-C constructs that could be expressed efficiently in eukaryotic cells. $P_{CMV}$-GBV-C-polyA gene cassettes were cloned into the HVS cosmid cos331 representing the N-terminal part of the HVS genome. Cosmid cos331 is part of a set of five cosmids coding for the whole genome of $HVS_{C488}$ (Figure 5-14). Transfection in Owl monkey kidney (OMK) cells leads to homologous recombination of HVS as well as to production of infectious $HVS_{GBV-C}$ chimeras. $HVS_{GBV-C}$ chimeras coding either for the N-terminal GBV-C proteins E1-E2-p5.6-NS2 or the nonstructural (NS) GBV-C proteins NS3-NS4A-NS4B and NS3-NS4A-NS4B-NS5A-NS5B were produced. Human T cell lines stable expressing the different GBV-C gene cassettes were generated by infection of CBL derived from 18 donors, by HVS as well as $HVS_{GBV-C}$ chimeras. HVS transformed T lymphocytes were cultivated in growth medium with or without IL-2 stimulation and expression of CD4, CCR5, and CXCR4 was monitored. In collaboration with the group of Prof. B. Fleckenstein and Ralf Müller, approximately 100 cell lines were generated. Whereas CCR5 and CXCR4 expression was not affected, IL-2 influenced differentiation of initial CD4/CD8 double positive CBL to CD4 or CD8 positive T cell lines. Taken together, 6 of 53 (11.3%) IL-2 treated, but 24 of 47 (51.1%) non-IL-2

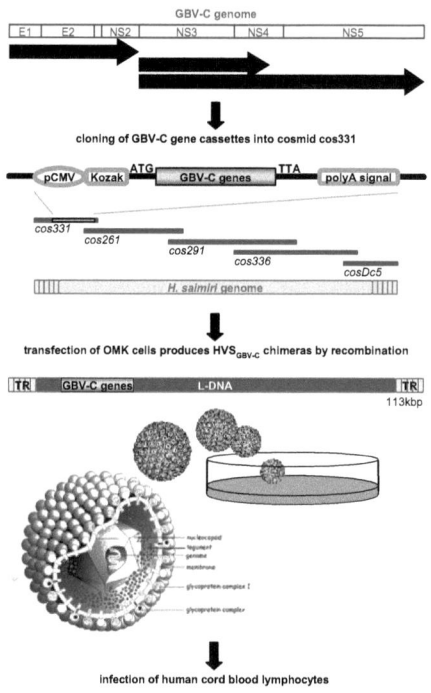

Figure 5-14: Generation of T cell lines stable expressing different GBV-C genes by infection of $HVS_{GBV-C}$ chimeras. GBV-C gene cassettes were cloned into cos331 and the entire cosmid set coding the whole $HVS_{C488}$ genome, was transfected in OMK cells. HVS reassembles via recombination and a cytopathic effect becomes visible. $HVS_{GBV-C}$ chimeras were harvested and used to infect and to transform human CBL.

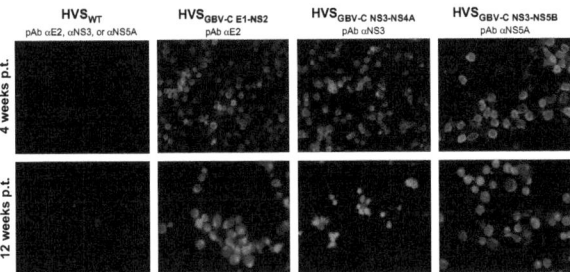

Figure 5-15: Protein expression in HVS$_{GBV-C}$ transformed T cell lines. Ongoing expression of GBV-C proteins in HVS$_{GBV-C}$ transformed CBL was monitored by immunofluorescence in relation to HVS$_{WT}$ (mock) transformed CBL. Permeabilized cells were stained with polyclonal antibodies directed against the E2, the NS3, or the NS5A protein, and labeled with anti-rabbit FITC antibodies.

treated cell lines differentiated to CD4 positive T cell lines until week 12 post transformation. Compared to HVS$_{GBV-C\ E1-NS2}$ (23.1%) transformed T cell lines, HVS$_{WT}$ (77.8%), HVS$_{GBV-C\ NS3-NS4B}$ (42.9%), and HVS$_{GBV-C\ NS3-NS5B}$ (61.1%) transformed T cell lines displayed an increased shift to CD4. Immunofluorescence using antibodies directed against the GBV-C E2, NS3, and NS5A protein proved the expression of at least one encoded GBV-C protein in each HVS$_{GBV-C}$ transformed cell line and thereby, ongoing expression of all GBV-C cassettes (Figure 5-15). To analyze the impact on HIV replication, CD4 positive T cell lines that displayed high GBV-C protein expression levels, were infected with HIV$_{WT}$ or HIV$_{PP}$. Comparable to GBV-C infected PBMC and T cell lines, expression of different GBV-C gene cassettes in HVS$_{GBV-C}$ transformed T cell lines suppressed the replication of CCR5- and CXCR4-tropic HIV isolates. Surprisingly, all GBV-C gene cassettes mediated an HIV-inhibitory effect suggesting that structural and nonstructural GBV-C proteins may be involved. Single round of infection assays using HIV$_{PP}$ corroborated these findings. In relation to HVS transformed cells, HIV$_{gp120}$ enveloped HIV$_{PP}$ were impaired on all HVS$_{GBV-C}$ transformed T cell lines. In contrast, VSV$_G$ envelope HIV$_{PP}$ were inhibited exclusively on T cell lines expressing the nonstructural GBV-C proteins. T cell lines expressing the structural GBV-C proteins (GBV-C$_{E1-NS2}$) did not affect the replication capacity of VSV$_G$ enveloped HIV$_{PP}$ (Figure 5-16). The data assume that the E1, E2, p5.6 or NS2 protein may interfere with the gp120/CD4-dependent entry of HIV, whereas one of the nonstructural GBV-C proteins (NS3, NS4A, NS4B, NS5A, NS5B) may influence later, cell entry independent HIV replication steps.

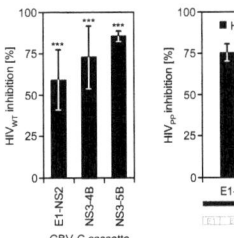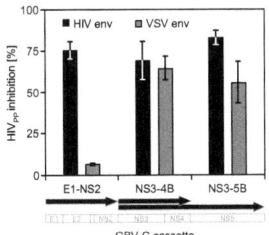

Figure 5-16: HIV inhibition on HVS$_{GBV-C}$ transformed T cell lines. HVS$_{WT}$ and HVS$_{GBV-C}$ transformed T cell lines were infected with clinical HIV isolates (left) and HIV$_{PP}$ enveloped either with HIV$_{gp120}$ or VSV$_G$ glycoproteins (right). Inhibition of HIV replication on HVS$_{GBV-C}$ transformed T cell lines was calculated in relation to HVS$_{WT}$ transformed cells. Grey arrows illustrate the GBV-C proteins that are expressed by the different HVS$_{GBV-C}$ transformed T cell lines.

### 5.3.3. Inhibition of different HIV Replication Steps by GB Virus C Proteins

To identify GBV-C proteins that are involved in HIV inhibition, each single GBV-C protein was expressed by the mammalian Tet expression system[106,107]. The vector system consists of a response plasmid that contains the gene of interest under the control of a tet-responsive element (TRE, pTRE2hyg) and an expression plasmid that codes for the tet-responsive

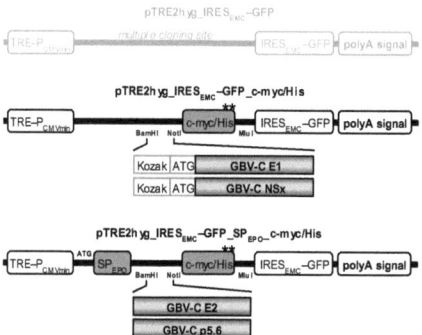

**Figure 5-17: Vectors for eukaryotic expression of GBV-C proteins.** The c-myc/His tag was cloned into pTRE2hyg_IRES$_{EMC}$-GFP to allow expression of c-myc/His proteins under the control of a tetracycline-responsive element (TRE). Additionally, the secretion signal sequence of erythropoietin (EPO) was cloned into pTRE2hyg_IRES$_{EMC}$–GFP_c-myc/His. The ORF of the E1 and the nonstructural proteins NS2, NS3, NS4A, NS4B, NS5A, and NS5B (NSx) were cloned into pTRE2hyg_IRES$_{EMC}$–GFP_c-myc/His. The ORF of the E2 and p5.6 protein was cloned into the expression vector pTRE2hyg_IRES$_{EMC}$–GFP_SP$_{EPO}$_c-myc/His.

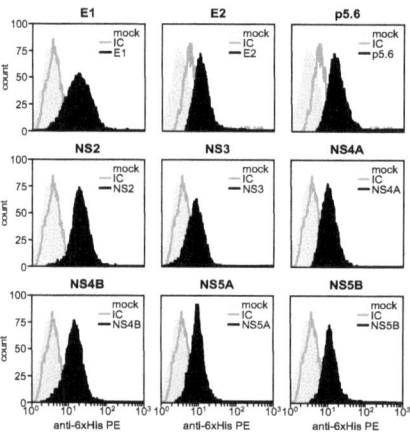

**Figure 5-18: Expression of GBV-C proteins in CEMx174$_{CCR5}$ Tet-Off cells.** One week post transfection, cells expressing the GBV-C_c-myc/His fusion proteins were analyzed by flow cytometry. Therefore, cells were harvested, washed, fixed with PFA, and permeabilized by saponine. Cells were stained either with isotype control antibodies (IC, grey line) or with PE conjugated anti-His antibodies (black line). Unstained cells that were transfected with the empty vector served as mock (filled grey area).

transcriptional activator (tTA, pTet-Off). After transfection of the response plasmid in a Tet-Off cell line, tTA binds to TRE and activates transcription in the absence of tetracycline or doxycycline. As tetracycline or doxycycline is added to the growth medium, transcription from the TRE driven promoter is turned off in a dose-dependent manner. To generate a stable Tet-Off T cell line, exponentially growing CEMx174$_{CCR5}$ cells were transfected with the pTet-Off plasmid using the Nucleofector™ technology (Lonza Cologne AG, Cologne). To enable efficient expression and post-translational processing of GBV-C surface proteins lacking an own signal peptide, the signal peptide sequence of erythropoietin (SP$_{EPO}$) was cloned into the eukaryotic tTA-responsive expression vector pTRE2hyg_IRES$_{EMC}$-GFP_c-myc/His. The ORF of each GBV-C protein was amplified from the clone AF121950 and cloned into pTRE2hyg_IRES$_{EMC}$-GFP_c-myc/His (E1, NS2, NS3, NS4A, NS4B, NS5A, NS5B) or pTRE2hyg_IRES$_{EMC}$-GFP_SP$_{EPO}$_c-myc/His (E1, p5.6), respectively (Figure 5-17). Next, expression constructs were transfected in CEMx174$_{CCR5}$ Tet-Off cells. Due to the IRES-GFP cassette that is regulated together with the respective GBV-C protein by the TRE-P$_{CMVmin}$ promoter, ongoing GBV-C protein expression could be monitored by green fluorescence. Protein expression was further analyzed by immunofluorescence and flow cytometry using PE conjugated anti-His antibodies (Figure 5-18). Antibodies directed against c-myc confirmed sufficient protein expression and were used to analyze the molecular weight of each fusion protein by SDS-Page and Western Blot analysis (data not shown). Cell toxicity assays revealed no differences between the individual proteins, even though, mock and GBV-C transfected cells showed an decreased proliferation rate in relation to native CEMx174$_{CCR5}$ cells.

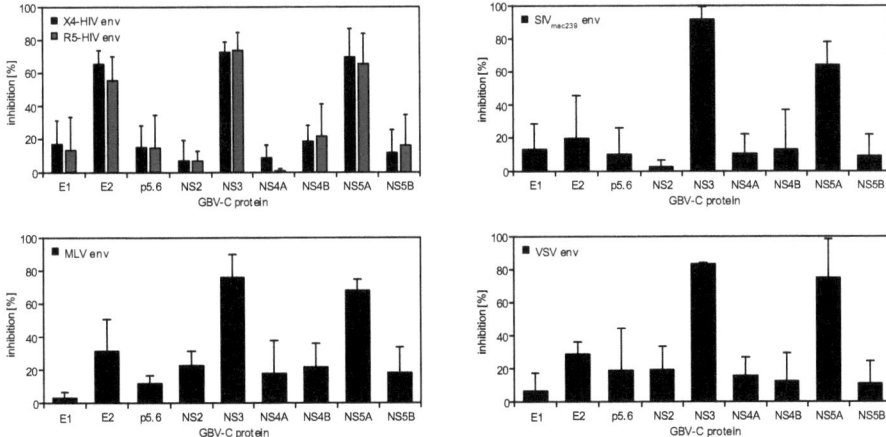

**Figure 5-19: Inhibition of HIV$_{PP}$ by the GBV-C proteins E2, NS3, and NS5A.** CEMx174$_{CCR5}$ Tet-Off cells expressing either the GBV-C protein E1, E2, p5.6, NS2, NS3, NS4A, NS4B, NS5A or NS5B, were infected with HIV-derived pseudoparticles bearing HIV, SIV$_{mac239}$, MLV, or VSV envelopes. Luciferase activity was measured in the cell lysates three days post infection and inhibition was calculated in relation to mock cells, which were transfected with the empty response vector. Columns represent average inhibition of at least three independent experiments performed in duplicates.

To investigate the HIV-inhibitory capacity of each single GBV-C protein, CEMx174$_{CCR5}$ Tet-Off cells expressing either the empty vector or the respective protein, were infected with HIV$_{PP}$. Whereas later HIV replication steps are identical, the cell entry mechanism of HIV$_{PP}$ depends of the expressed viral envelope. HIV$_{gp120}$ and SIV$_{gp130}$ enveloped HIV$_{PP}$ infect target cells via receptor mediated fusion. Whereas, HIV$_{gp120}$ induces binding to CD4 and CCR5 or CXCR4, SIV$_{gp130}$ mediates infection via binding to Bob or Bonzo. MLV$_{gp80}$ enveloped HIV$_{PP}$ bind to Pit and infect cells by receptor mediated endocytosis. VSV$_G$ enveloped HIV$_{PP}$ elude a receptor binding mechanism and infect target cells by endocytosis and acidification of the endosome[48,71,80,269,295]. Whereas the GBV-C E2 protein inhibited the gp120/CD4-dependent HIV entry mechanism, the NS3 and the NS5A protein impaired HIV$_{PP}$ with different viral envelopes suggesting that HIV replication steps other than entry may be affected (Figure 5-19).

## 5.4. Identification of the GB Virus C E2 Protein as HIV Entry Inhibitor

Expression of the GBV-C proteins E1, E2, p5.6, and NS2 inhibited HIV$_{PP}$. Furthermore, it was postulated that the E2 protein decreases the expression of CCR5[195]. Since reduced co-receptor expression may impair binding and fusion of CCR5-HIV, it should be evaluated, if structural GBV-C proteins and in particular the E2 protein may be responsible for the observed HIV-inhibitory effect in cell culture.

### 5.4.1. HIV Suppression by Transfection of RNA encoding the GB Virus C Glycoproteins

Expression of the N-terminal GBV-C gene cassette E1-N2 in CBL by a rhadinovirus based vector system as well as expression of the GBV-C E2 protein in CEMx174$_{CCR5}$ cells using the Tet-Off system, inhibited HIV replication in cell culture. To prove the involvement of the

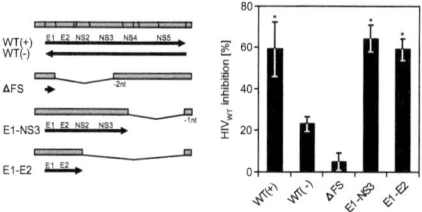

Figure 5-20: Inhibition of HIV$_{WT}$ by transfection of RNA encoding the GBV-C envelope proteins. PBMC were transfected with full-length RNA of the GBV-C clone AF121950 (WT), RNA of a frame shift mutant (ΔFS) or mutants coding the E1-E2-p5.6-NS2-NS3 (E1-NS3) or E1-E2 (E1-E2) protein prior HIV$_{WT}$ infection was performed. Yellow bars illustrate nucleotide sequences, black arrows ORF. Columns represent average inhibition of three independent experiments.

structural GBV-C proteins in HIV suppression by another approach, fresh isolated PBMC were transfected with full length plus- or minus-strand RNA derived from the infectious GBV-C clone AF121950 or different GBV-C deletion mutants. Hereby, each RNA was flanked by the natural 5' and 3' UTR of GBV-C including the autologous IRES. Transfection of plus-strand RNA encoding either the whole GBV-C proteom (WT(+)) or the proteins E1-E2-p5.6-NS2-NS3 or E1-E2, led to transient protein expression, which could be confirmed by immunofluorescence using anti-E2 antibodies. In contrast, post transfection of RNA derived from a frameshift mutant (ΔFS) or full length minus-strand RNA (WT(-)) that served as negative controls, no expression of GBV-C proteins could be observed (data not shown). Three to four days post transfection, cells were harvested and HIV$_{WT}$ infection was performed and monitored by p24 release into the supernatant. In comparison to mock transfected cells, expression of the GBV-C proteins E1, E2, p5.6, and NS2 led to significant inhibition of HIV replication. In contrast, expression of minus-strand RNA (WT(-)) and RNA of ΔFS that codes just the first part of the E1 protein, failed to suppress HIV (Figure 5-20). The data corroborate previous findings and reveal that the GBV-C E2, p5.6 or NS2 protein are involved in GBV-C mediated HIV inhibition.

### 5.4.2. Expression, Purification, and Characterization of GB Virus C E2(340)-Fc Fusion Proteins

The GBV-C glycoproteins E1 and E2 are encoded in the N-terminal part of the GBV-C genome and it is suggested that these proteins play a crucial role in GBV-C entry and fusion. It has been shown that binding of the 40S ribosomal subunit to the IRES located in the 5' UTR, initiates translation of the GBV-C polyprotein in a cap-independent manner[262]. A signal peptide within the E1 amino acid sequence refers the nascent viral polyprotein to the granular endoplasmatic reticulum (rER), where the viral glycoproteins are released by host-cell signal peptidases. E1 and E2 assemble as non-covalent heterodimers. Both proteins are type I transmembrane proteins, with N-terminal ectodomains and a short C-terminal transmembrane domain that is formed by two stretches of hydrophobic residues and that plays an important role in membrane anchoring, ER localization, and heterodimer assembly (Figure 5-21). To investigate the impact of the GBV-C E2 protein on HIV replication, a soluble form of the E2 protein was cloned. In line with the nomenclature of the GBV-C isolate AF121950, the E2 protein consists of 388 amino acids, coded by the nucleotides 1164-2328 (amino acids 330-717 of the GBV-C polyprotein). The transmembrane domain of the E2 protein is formed by the amino acids 340-384. To generate truncated versions of the E2 protein derived from the GBV-C clones AF121950 and HGU44402 as well as of clinical GBV-C isolates, respective sequences lacking the amino acids 341-388 of the E2 protein were amplified by high fidelity

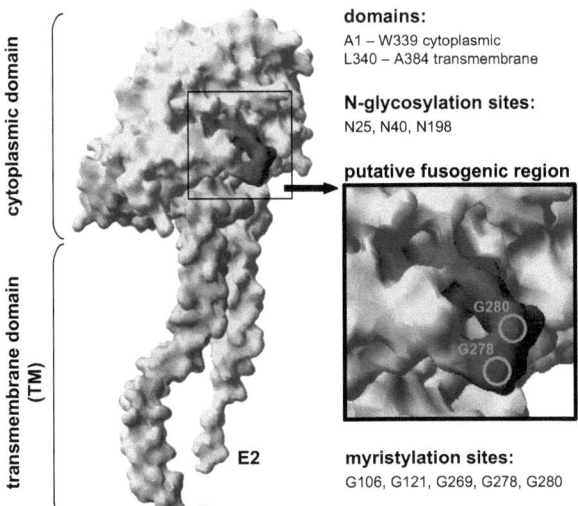

Figure 5-21: Model of the GBV-C envelope proteins E1 and E2. The I-TASSER server was used to calculate a three-dimensional model of the E1 (grey) and E2 (yellow) protein of the GBV-C isolate AF121950. Each protein consists of a cytoplasma and a transmembrane domain. The globular E2 domain is formed by the amino acids (aa) 1–339. The transmembrane domain is formed by the aa340–384. The E2 protein offers three glycosylation and five myristoylation sites that may play an important role in protein-protein interactions as well as cell signaling processes. The close up displays the putative GBV-C E2 fusion peptide (petrol) and two myristoylation sites (green circle) that may be involved in GBV-C cell binding to the currently unknown cellular receptor.

polymerase chain reaction and cloned into the eukaryotic expression vector pCEP4-Fc. Hereby, the N-terminus of the E2 protein was fused to the signal peptide of the murine IgG$_\kappa$ V-J2-C chain. The C-terminal transmembrane domain was replaced with the human IgG$_1$ Fc domain, a c-myc as well as a polyhistidine tag to enhance the yield of secreted E2(340)-Fc fusion protein and to simplify detection and purification. The use of an eukaryotic expression system assured the N-linked glycosylation pattern and other posttranslational features of the E2 protein. 293T cells were transfected with pCEP4-Fc and pCEP4-E2(340)-Fc expression vectors Stable transfected clones were selected and protein expression was monitored by ELISA. For this purpose, cell lysates and cell culture supernatants of respective clones were incubated with the biotinylated monoclonal murine anti-E2 antibody M5 (Roche Diagnostics, Penzberg) and transferred into a streptavidine coated 96-well plate, to capture recombinant E2 protein. Polyclonal rabbit anti-E2 antibodies (Jack Stapleton, University of Iowa) were added and bound E2 protein was detected by HRP conjugated goat anti-rabbit IgG antibodies (Dako, Hamburg). Alternatively, recombinant E2(340)-Fc fusion proteins were detected directly by HRP conjugated rabbit anti-human IgG antibodies (Dako, Hamburg). Soluble E2(340)-Fc fusion proteins derived from the GBV-C clones AF121950 and HGU044402 as well as the clinical GBV-C isolates 440, 10750, D1007, D1108, and D1902 could be detected in cell lysates and supernatants of transfected 293T cells. In contrast, full length E2 could be detected just in the cell lysates. Intracellular staining by fluorescein isothiocyanate (FITC) conjugated antibodies directed against human IgG (Dako, Hamburg) or the E2 protein (Jackson IR, West Grove), corroborated the expression of E2(340)-Fc fusion proteins and of the sole Fc fragment (Figure 5-22). In addition, protein expression was proved by western blot (data not shown). E2(340)-Fc and sole Fc fragment containing supernatants were collected, filtered through a 0.22μm filter, and purified by affinity chromatography. Thereby, the high binding affinity of the Fc fragment to Protein A was used. Cell-free supernatants of E2(340)-Fc and sole Fc fragment expressing cells were subjected to a HiTrap Protein A FF column (GE Healthcare, Munich) with a flow

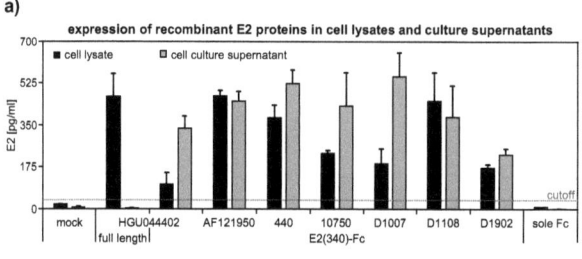

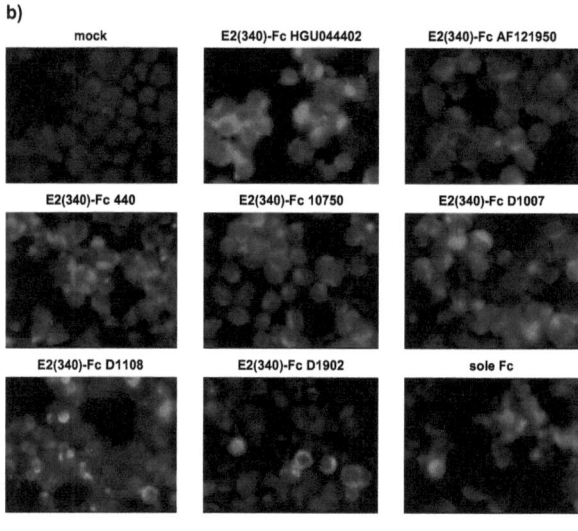

Figure 5-22: Expression of GBV-C E2(340)-Fc fusion proteins in 293T cells. a) To determine the concentration of full length E2 and truncated E2(340)-Fc proteins in supernatants and cell lysates of stable transfected 293T cells, a quantitative ELISA using polyclonal rabbit anti-E2 antibodies (Jack Stapleton, University of Iowa) was performed. Efficient expression of full length E2 derived from the GBV-C clone HGU044402 as well as of recombinant GBV-C E2(340)-Fc fusion proteins derived from the clones HGU044402 and AF121950 and of the clinical GBV-C isolates 440, 10750, D1007, D1108, and D1902 was monitored. Supernatants and lysates of mock cells and cells expressing the sole Fc fragment, served as negative controls. b) Protein expression was visualized by immunofluorescence. 293T cells were harvested one month post transfection. Cells were fixed with PFA and permeabilized by saponine and recombinant Fc fusion proteins were stained using FITC conjugated anti-human IgG antibodies (Dako, Hamburg). Green: intra and extra cellular staining of the E2(340)-Fc fusion proteins and the sole Fc fragment, blue: DAPI staining of the cell nuclei.

rate of one milliliter per minute. Column bound proteins were eluted by 0.1M citric acid using a pH gradient ranging from 5 to 3. Fractions were neutralized immediately by adding 1M Tris HCl (pH 9). Protein containing fractions were screened by western blot. Selected fractions were pooled and elution buffer was changed against PBS. Protein concentrations were determined and aliquots were stored at -80°C until use. SDS-Page, Coomassie staining, and western blot analysis using monoclonal anti-E2 antibodies as well as polyclonal anti-human IgG antibodies, were performed to analyze size and purity of the proteins in the respective elution fraction. Whereas the sole Fc_c-myc/His fragment formed a single distinct protein band with an

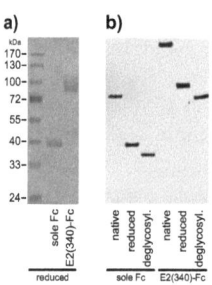

Figure 5-23: Characterization of Fc fusion proteins. a) To analyze purification efficiency and molecular weight of the sole Fc fragment as well as of the E2(340)-Fc fusion protein derived from the GBV-C clone AF121950, protein samples were analyzed by SDS-Page and Coomassie staining. b) Additionally, sole Fc and E2(340)-Fc fusion proteins were investigated by western blot analysis under non-reducing (native) and reducing condition and stained by HRP conjugated rabbit anti-human IgG antibodies (Dako, Hamburg). To investigate the glycosylation pattern, 2µg of the purified sole Fc fragment as well as of the E2(340)-Fc protein were denatured for 10 minutes at 95°C in the presence of 0.5% SDS and 1% ß-Mercaptoethanol. 2U of N-GlycosidaseF (PNGaseF, New England Biolabs, Frankfurt/Main), 2µl of NP40 (10%), and 2µl of 0.5M sodium phosphate (pH 7.5) were added and incubated for 2 hours at 37°C prior samples were analyzed by SDS-PAGE and western blot.

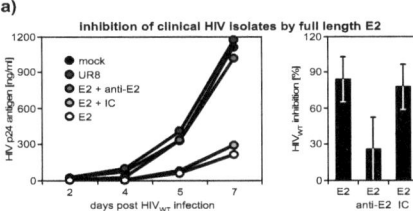 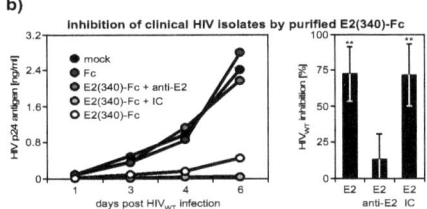

**Figure 5-24: Inhibition of HIV$_{WT}$ and HIV$_{PP}$ by recombinant GBV-C E2 proteins.** To investigate the impact of recombinant GBV-C E2 protein on HIV replication, PBMC were incubated either with **a)** cell lysate with full length E2 or **b)** with purified E2(340)-Fc fusion protein lacking the transmembrane domaine. A cell lysate containing the urokinase receptor 8 (UR8) and purified Fc fragment served as negative controls. To prove the specificity of the E2-mediated effect, recombinant E2 proteins were preincubated with anti-E2 or the respective isotype control (IC) antibodies for one hour at 4°C. E2 as well as antibody treated E2 proteins were used to stimulate PBMC for one hour at 4°C. Post incubation, cells were washed and cultivated for 24–48 hours prior HIV infection was performed. Supernatants were collected at different time points and p24 antigen concentration was quantified. Line charts display representative single experiments. Columns represent the average inhibition of at least three independent experiments calculated in relation to mock.

apparent molecular weight of 40kDa, the E2(340)-Fc fusion protein showed a protein band corresponding to a molecular size of 95kDa. PNGaseF deglycosilation, which cleaves N-linked carbohydrates, led to a motility shift of E2(340)-Fc fusions protein of ~20kDa. This is in agreement with three putative consensus glycosylation sites and the predicted size of the polypeptide backbone of 74kDa. Western blot analysis under non-reducing conditions suggested that the hinge region within the Fc mediates expression of both, Fc and E2(340)-Fc, as non-covalent bound homodimers (Figure 5-23). To investigate the HIV-inhibitory capacity of recombinant E2, PBMC were incubated with the sole Fc as well as with full length and truncated GBV-C E2 protein prior HIV$_{WT}$ infection was performed. Indeed, full length E2 as well as truncated E2(340)-Fc impaired the replication of clinical HIV isolates in a comparable manner. Preincubation of recombinant E2 with anti-E2 antibodies abolished the inhibitory effect and proved the specificity of GBV-C E2 mediated HIV inhibition (Figure 5-24). Artificial effects due to cell toxicity could be excluded, since E2 stimulated and untreated PBMC displayed similar cell proliferation rates (data not shown). For further investigation, single round of infection assays using HIV$_{PP}$ bearing envelopes of CCR5- and CXCR4-tropic HIV isolates or envelopes of heterologous viruses, were performed. In brief, CEMx174 or CEMx174$_{CCR5}$ cells were incubated with different amounts of full length E2, truncated E2(340)-Fc fusion proteins or of the sole Fc fragment prior infection with HIV$_{gp120}$ or VSV$_G$ enveloped HIV$_{PP}$ was performed. Three days later, luciferase activity was measured and suppression of HIV$_{PP}$ was calculated in relation to PBS stimulated cells. Again, full length E2 of the GBV-C clone HGU44402 as well as E2(340)-Fc fusion proteins derived from HIV-inhibitory (AF121950, 10750) or intermediated GBV-C isolates (D1902) to inhibit HIV$_{gp120}$ enveloped HIV$_{PP}$. In contrast, E2(340)-Fc proteins derived from HIV-non-inhibitory GBV-C isolates (D1007, D1108) and the sole Fc fragment did not. Interestingly, none of the E2 proteins were able to inhibit VSV$_G$ enveloped HIV$_{PP}$ (Figure 5-25a). Specificity of GBV-C E2 mediated inhibition of HIV entry could be shown by preincubation of recombinant E2 with anti-E2 antibodies that abolished the inhibitory effect (Figure 5-25b). Taken together, the data suggested a causal relation between the observed suppression of HIV entry by incubation with recombinant E2 protein and inhibition of HIV entry by infection with clinical GBV-C isolates.

To compare the HIV-inhibitory potency of different E2(340)-Fc fusion proteins, the average concentration of each recombinant E2 protein that reduce the activity of HIVPP by 50% ($IC_{50}$), was determined in relation to the sole Fc fragment. $IC_{50}$ of E2(340)-Fc fusion proteins derived from HIV-inhibitory GBV-C isolates correspond to approximately 6nM (Figure 5-25c). Since the amino acids E143 and T204 were mutated exclusively in E2 protein of HIV-non-inhibitory GBV-C isolates (Figure 5-8), HIV-inhibitory capacity of the respective parenteral E2 sequences was investigated. Therefore, CEMx174$_{CCR5}$ cells were incubated with overlapping peptides

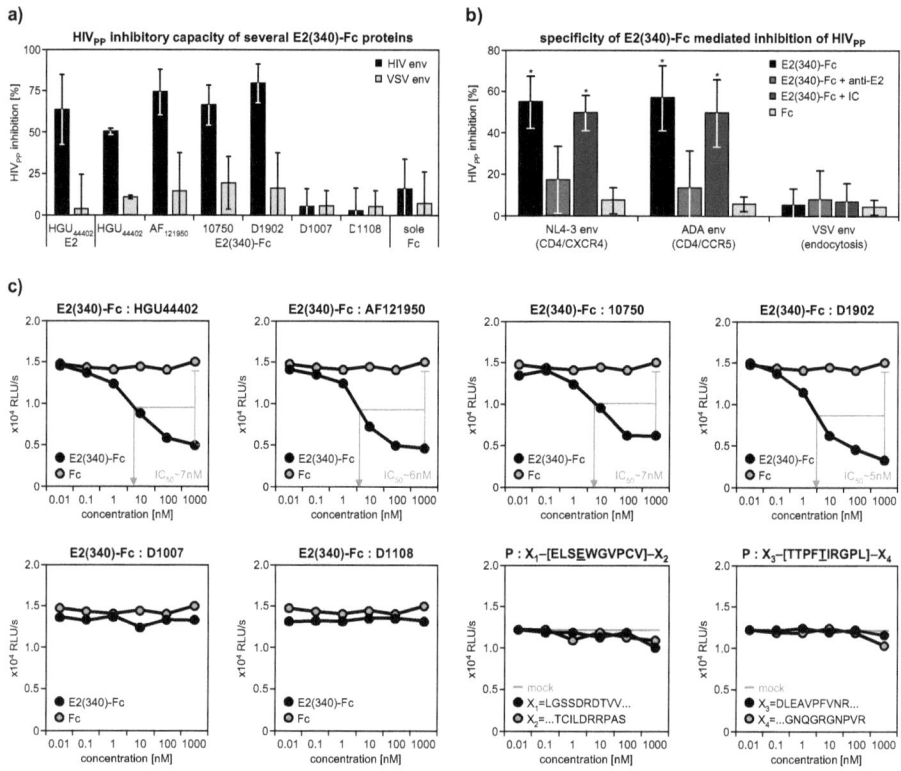

**Figure 5-25: E2(340)-Fc fusion proteins of HIV-inhibitory GBV-C isolates inhibit the gp120/CD4-dependent HIV entry mechanism.** a) CEMx174$_{CCR5}$ cells were incubated with 15nM of the sole Fc fragment or of the E2(340)-Fc fusion protein derived from several GBV-C isolates with different HIV-inhibitory phenotypes: inhibitory (AF121950, 10750), intermediate (D1902), and HIV-non-inhibitory (D1007, D1108). E2 stimulation was performed for 1 hour at 4°C prior cells were washed and cultivated for 48 hours. Single round of infection assays using CXCR4- and CCR5-tropic HIV$_{gp120}$ as well as VSV$_G$ enveloped HIV$_{PP}$ were performed. Luciferase activity was measured 72 hours later. Columns represent the average HIV$_{PP}$ inhibition of at least two independent experiments performed in triplicates. b) Specificity was proved by preincubation of E2(340)-Fc derived from the HIV-inhibitory GBV-C clone AF121950, with anti-E2 antibodies or respective isotype control (IC) antibodies prior incubation of CEMx174$_{CCR5}$ cells and single round of infection assay was performed. Columns represent the average inhibition of HIV$_{PP}$ of at least three independent experiments performed in triplicates. c) CEMx174$_{CCR5}$ cells were incubated with increasing amounts of the respective E2(340)-Fc fusion protein or the sole Fc fragment prior cells were subjected to single round of infection assays. Additionally, CEMx174$_{CCR5}$ cells were incubated with overlapping 20mer peptides derived from the HIV-inhibitory GBV-C clone AF121950 harboring the aa E143 (LGSSDRDTVV[ELSEWGVPCV], [ELSEWGVPCV]TCILDRRPAS) or T204 (DLEAVPFVNR[TTPFTIRGPL], [TTPFTIRGPL]GNQGRGNPVR) that are mutated in the E2 protein of HIV-non-neutralizing GBV-C isolates.

corresponding to the E2 protein sequence of the GBV-C isolate AF121950, prior infection assays using HIV$_{gp120}$ enveloped HIV$_{PP}$ were performed. Each overlapping 20mer peptide contained either E143 (LGSSDRDTVVELS<u>E</u>WGVPCV, ELS<u>E</u>WGVPCVTCILDRRPAS) or T204 (DLEAVPFVNRTTPF<u>T</u>IRGPL, TTPF<u>T</u>IRGPLGNQGRGNPVR). In contrast to the recombinant E2(340)-Fc fusion protein of AF121950, none of the peptides was able to supress HIV$_{PP}$ in a comparable manner (Figure 5-25c). The data suggest that E143 and T204 did not affect the HIV-inhibitory capacity of GBV-C E2. Thus, it is unlikely that E143K/H or T204A is responsible for the distinct HIV-inhibitory phenotypes of clinical GBV-C isolates. Nevertheless, the data prove the interference of GBV-C E2 with the gp120/CD4-dependent cell entry of HIV. Additionally, it could be demonstrated that some GBV-C isolates harbor E2 proteins that do not have this HIV-inhibitory ability.

### 5.4.3. Mechanism of GB Virus C E2-mediated HIV Inhibition

Incubation of HIV target cells with recombinant GBV-C E2 protein inhibits HIV$_{WT}$ as well as HIV$_{gp120}$ enveloped HIV$_{PP}$ independent of the co-receptor tropism of respective HIV particles. Since inhibition of early HIV replication steps depends on the expression of CD4, CCR5, and CXCR4, PBMC were incubated with GBV-C E2 and receptor expression was monitored by flow cytometry. In addition, cell surface expression of CD81, the suggested cellular receptor for GBV-C[195], was investigated. Hereby, no changes of CD81, CD4, and CXCR4 surface density due to E2 stimulation could be observed. In contrast, the percentage of CCR5 positive cells was significantly reduced on E2 stimulated cells. Both, full length E2 as well as truncated E2(340)-Fc fusion protein mediated a significant and dose-dependent down regulation of CCR5. Preincubation with E2-directed antibodies neutralized the observed effect (Figure 5-26). Supernatants of E2 stimulated cells were collected and concentration of RANTES, MIP1alpha, MIP-1beta, and SDF-1 was quantified by ELISA. Interestingly, recombinant E2 induces exclusively the beta-chemokines RANTES, MIP-1alpha, and MIP-1beta. In contrast, induction of the alpha-chemokine SDF-1 could be observed (Figure 5-27a). Noteworthy, the observed correlation between chemokine secretion and CCR5 down regulation strongly depended on the PBMC donor. Therefore, an alternative fluorescence based muliplex ELISA (Luminex, Coley Pharmaceutical, Cologne) was performed. In this setting, induction of MIP-1alpha, MIP-1beta,

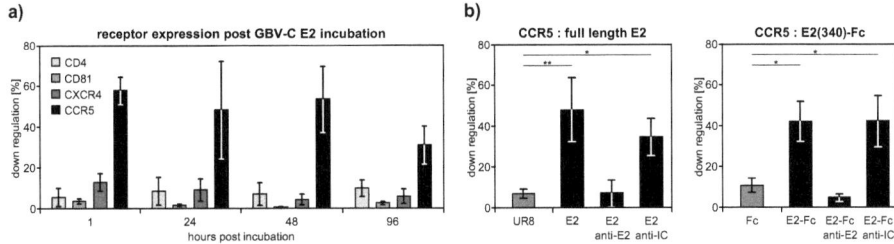

Figure 5-26: Down regulation of CCR5 surface expression by recombinant GBV-C E2 proteins. a) PBMC were incubated for 1 hour at 4°C with PBS or recombinant GBV-C E2 proteins, washed, and cultivated for up to 96 hours. At different time points, cells were harvested and expression of CD4, CD81, CXCR4, and CCR5 was analyzed. b) Specificity could be proved by preincubation with anti-E2 antibodies that abolished the HIV-inhibitory effect of recombinant E2. In contrast preincubation with respective isotype control (IC) antibodies or cell lysate containing a recombinant form of the urokinase receptor 8 (UR8, mock) as well as with purified sole Fc fragment had no effect and served as negative controls.

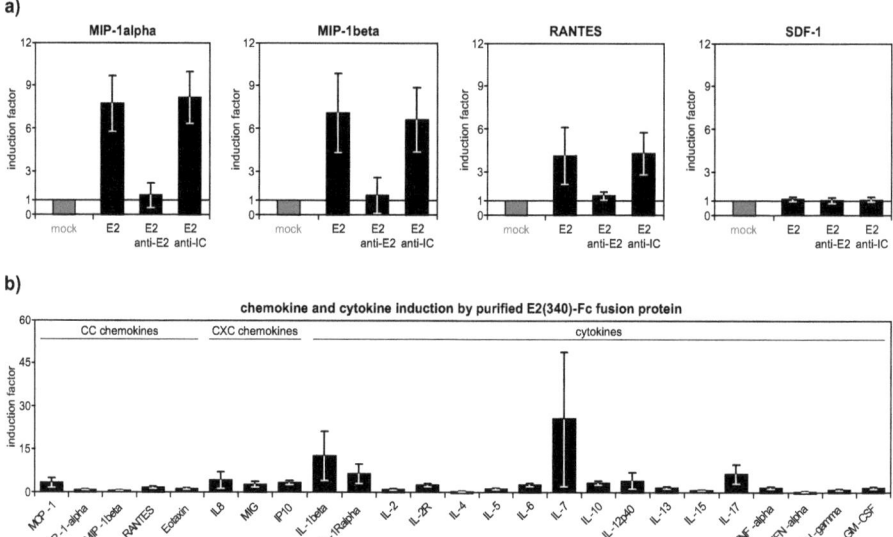

**Figure 5-27: Chemokine and cytokine induction by recombinant GBV-C E2 proteins. a)** PBMC were incubated with cell lysate containing full length E2, washed, and cultivated as described earlier. Supernatants were collected at five time points (1h – 7days) and concentration of MIP-1alpha, MIP-1beta, RANTES, and SDF-1 was determined by ELISA. Induction factors were calculated in relation to untreated cells. Columns represent average induction factors of at least two independent experiments. Factors higher than one indicate stimulation of chemokine secretion. Specificity of the observed effect could be demonstrated by preincubation of recombinant E2 with anti-E2 antibodies that abolished the effect. **b)** PBMC of five different blood donors were incubated with E2(340)-F, washed, and concentration of different chemo- and cytokines was quantified by the Luminex multiplex-ELISA (Coley Pharmaceutical, Cologne)

and RANTES could not be confirmed. Additionally, increased concentrations of IL-1beta and IL-7 could be detected in supernatants of E2(340)-Fc stimulated PBMC. IL-1beta is a proinflammatory cytokine that plays a crucial role in triggering the immune response during various diseases. It has been shown that IL-1beta contribute to cellular inflammation and is an important mediator during systemic as well as local inflammation. In contrast, IL-7 is a pleiotropic cytokine that plays a major role in T cell homeostasis and participates in humoral inflammation. Since just a moderate secretion of IL-1beta and IL-7 could be observed, an impact on E2/HIV interference could be excluded (Figure 5-27b). To further investigate, if cell bound GBV-C E2 protein masks cellular receptors, PBMC and several cell lines with distinct receptor profiles were incubated with full-length E2 and truncated E2(340)-Fc. E2 cell binding ability and surface expression of CD81, CCR5, CXCR4, CD3, CD4, CD8, and CD19 was examined by flow cytometry. Thereby, efficient binding of recombinant GBV-C E2 to PBMC, CEMx174, Molt-4, and Hela cells could be observed. Again, specificity could be proved by preincubation of recombinant E2 with anti-E2 antibodies that led to a reduced binding affinity. In contrast, pretreatment of E2 with isotype control antibodies had no effect. In contrast, recombinant E2 did not bound to Jurkat and Daudi cells. Furthermore, since all cell lines express high amounts of CD81, the data imply that CD81 is not mandatory to mediated E2 cell binding. Comparison of the receptor expression profile of E2 bound and non-E2-bound cells revealed that neither the B (CD19) and T cell receptors (CD3, CD4, CD8) nor the HIV

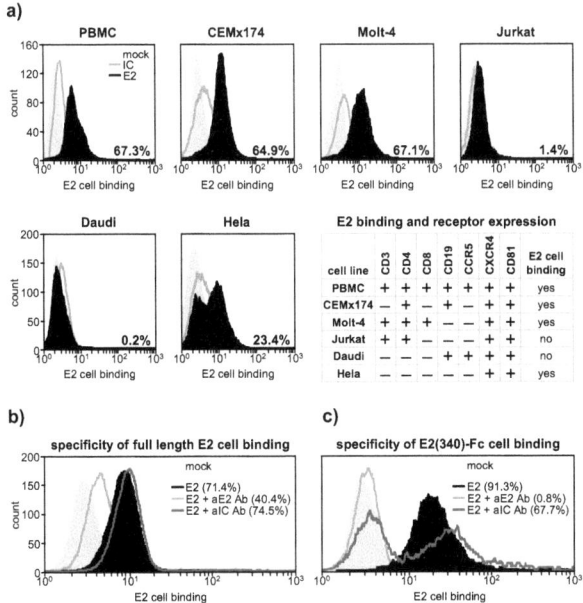

Figure 5-28: Recombinant GBV-C E2 proteins bind to human cells. a) PBMC, B and T cell lines (CEMx174: B/T, Molt-4: T, Jurkat: T, Daudi: B cell line), and Hela cells were incubated with recombinant E2. Cell bound E2 was stained using the murine anti-E2 antibody M5 (black) or respective isotype control (IC) antibodies as well as FITC conjugated anti-mouse antibodies. E2 cell binding was quantified by flow cytometry in relation to unstained cells (mock). For each cell type a representative experiment is shown. Percent values correspond to the average amount of E2 bound cells calculated of at least two experiments. The table summarizes the E2 cell binding affinity and the presence of several cell surface receptors. Specificity of E2 cell binding was proved by preincubation of b) full length E2 and c) E2(340)-Fc with anti-E2 or IC antibodies prior binding assay on Molt-4 cells was performed.

co-receptors (CCR5, CXCR4) are necessary of efficient E2 cell binding. Moreover, the E2 protein did not decrease the number of CCR5 positive cells by a masking effect (Figure 5-28). Since the E2 protein has a high affinity to CEMx174, Molt-4, and Hela cells that do not express CCR5 and since the E2 protein did not bind to Jurkat and Daudi cells that express high levels of CXCR4, it could be exclude that CCR5 or CXCR4 represent the main or exclusive GBV-C receptor. Therefore, it is unlikely that E2 mediates HIV entry inhibition by an interference mechanism affecting HIV receptor binding.

## 5.5. Induction of HIV-neutralizing Antibodies by GB Virus C

GBV-C prevalence is higher in HIV patients than in the general population. Up to 70% of HIV positives have been exposed to GBV-C and approximately one third are positive for anti-E2 antibodies that serve as marker for a previous infection[277,288,288]. Epidemiological studies demonstrate that not only GBV-C viremia, but also anti-E2 antibodies are associated with prolonged survival of HIV patients[287,308]. To investigate, if a mimikry phenomenon between GBV-C and HIV exists and to analyze wether antibodies directed against the E2 protein may crossreact with HIV particles and inhibit HIV, neutralization assays should be performed.

### 5.5.1. Screening for anti-E2 Antibodies Positive Blood Donors

To investigate the role of anti-E2 antibodies in HIV binding and suppression, sera from healthy HIV, HCV, HBV as well as GBV-C RNA negative volunteers were collected and screened for the presence of anti-E2 antibodies using the µPate anti-HGenv ELISA (Roche Diagnostics, Penzberg). Four of 19 volunteers were tested positive for anti-E2 antibodies (Figure 5-29a).

The prevalence of anti-E2 antibodies (21%) was slightly higher than in the literature[146,174,201]. To confirm the specificity of anti-E2 reactive samples and to exclude that positive ELISA results were caused by other serum proteins, IgG fractions were purified by Protein A/G affinity chromatography. Sera were centrifuged, filtered through a 0.22µm filter, and loaded onto a Protein A/G column with a flow rate of one milliliter per minute. Unspecific bound proteins were removed by rinsing the column with five column volumes of wash buffer. Human IgG were eluted at pH 3.1 and pH 2.7 and neutralized immediately to pH 7 by adding 1M Tris-HCl (pH 9). Protein concentrations were determined and purity was investigated by SDS-polyacrylamide gel electrophoresis (PAGE, data not shown). To verify specificity and reactivity of antibody preparations, recombinant E2 protein was expressed and prepared as described earlier[278] and spotted onto PVDF membranes prior comparable amounts of anti-E2 positive and negative human IgG fractions were added. A set of eight murine monoclonal anti-E2 antibodies[250] served as positive control. Polyclonal IgG preparations of anti-E2 positive blood donors displayed an E2-specific reactivity. Comparable to the eight monoclonal anti-E2 antibodies detecting conformational (M3, M5, M11, M13, M17, M19, M30) as well as linear epitops (M6) of the GBV-C E2 protein, the human polyclonal anti-E2 positive IgG fractions recognized both, conformational as well as linear epitopes on native and/or denatured E2, respectively (Figure 5-29b). To narrow down, which subclass of human IgG features the main reactivity against the GBV-C E2 protein, the different binding affinities of Protein A and G to $IgG_1$, $IgG_2$, $IgG_3$, and $IgG_4$, were used. Whereas Protein G binds all human IgG subclasses with comparable efficiencies and allows purification of the whole IgG fraction, Protein A binds exclusively to $IgG_1$, $IgG_2$, and $IgG_4$ and enables separation of the $IgG_3$ subfraction that remains in the flow through. The reactivity of purified $IgG_{1,2,3,4}$, $IgG_{1,2,4}$, and

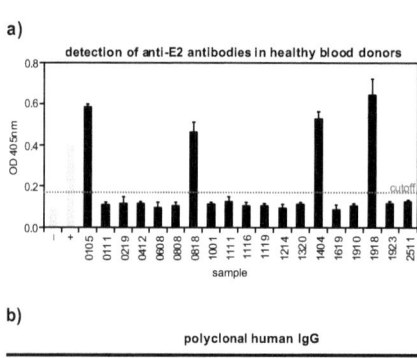

**Figure 5-29: Screening for GBV-C anti-E2 antibodies.** Healthy blood donors were screened for anti-E2 antibodies. **a)** Four (0105, 0818, 1404, 1918) of 19 serum samples tested positive for GBV-C anti-E2 antibodies using the µPlate HGenv ELISA (Roche Diagnostic, Penzberg) according to the manufactures protocol. Columns represent the average reactivity of the respective serum sample determined by two independent experiments. **b)** Positive samples were corroborated by immunoblot analysis. To minimize unspecific serum effects, IgG fractions of anti-E2 positive and negative blood donors were purified by Protein A/G affinity chromatography. A set of eight monoclonal antibodies raised in mice were also tested to exclude that GBV-C E2 unrelated antibodies are responsible for the observed reactivity. Recombinant GBV-C E2 protein was eukaryotic expressed and prepared as described earlier. Native and boiled E2 protein (10mM ß-Mercaptoethanol, 99°C) was spotted onto an equilibrated PVDF membrane. The membrane was blocked and each protein dot was incubated with 100ng of purified polyclonal human IgG or monoclonal murine anti-E2 antibodies. E2 binding was detected either with rabbit anti-human HRP or with goat anti-mouse HRP prior the blot was developed by enhanced chemiluminescence peroxidase solution. Detection of native and denatured (99°C) E2 proteins revealed that human anti-E2 antibodies are directed against conformational and linear epitopes of the GBV-C E2 protein.

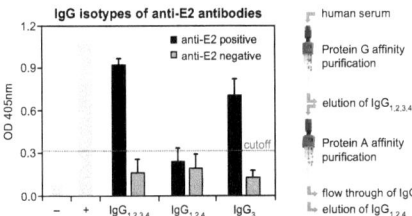

Figure 5-30: Determent of the IgG isotype of human anti-E2 antibodies. Anti-E2 positive and negative IgG fractions were purified by Protein G and Protein A affinity chromatography. Due to the lack of efficient IgG$_3$ binding by Protein A, IgG$_3$ could be separated from IgG$_{1,2,4}$ and remained in the flow through. The µPlate anti-HGenv ELISA was used to determine the reactivity of the respective IgG fraction. Each column represents the average extinction of the IgG subfractions according to the anti-E2 antibody status of the blood donor.

IgG$_3$ of four anti-E2 positive and four anti-E2 negative blood donors were tested using the µPLATE anti-HGenv ELISA. Comparable to previous findings, neither sera nor purified IgG fractions of anti-E2 negative volunteers recognized the E2 antigen. In contrast, purified IgG$_{1,2,3,4}$ as well as the IgG$_3$ subfraction of anti-E2 positive blood donors were reactive. Interestingly, IgG$_{1,2,4}$ preparations lacking the IgG$_3$ subfraction, were not able to detect the GBV-C E2 protein suggesting that human anti-E2 antibodies represent predominantly, but not exclusively, IgG of subclass three (Figure 5-30).

## 5.5.2. HIV Neutralization by anti-E2 Antibodies

To prove the hypothesis, whether anti-E2 antibodies suppress HIV, neutralization activity of GBV-C RNA negative, but anti-E2 positive sera was evaluated. Indeed, anti-E2 positive sera provided a neutralization activity, which was not seen with anti-E2 negative sera or anti-E2 positive sera, when the IgG fraction was removed (data not shown). Considering that these neutralization activity was mediated by anti-E2 positive IgG, polyclonal IgG preparations of four anti-E2 positive and negative donors were tested in neutralization assays on PBMC using HIV$_{WT}$ isolates. All IgG preparations with detectable amounts of anti-E2 antibodies had a broad and potent neutralization activity against a variety of HIV$_{WT}$ isolates representing different clades of group M and O. IC$_{50}$ values ranged from 0.01µg/ml to 6µg/ml. Hereby the potency was not influenced by the coreceptor tropism of the respective HIV isolate. To prove that the observed effect is mediated by anti-E2 antibodies, the set of eight murine monoclonal anti-E2 antibodies were also tested using the same HIV virus panel. Within the same assay, the HIV-inhibitory potency of anti-E2 antibodies was compared with the inhibitory potentcy of the human monoclonal HIV-neutralizing antibodies 2G12, F425B4e8, and 2F5. Whereas 2G12 and F425B4e8 binds to HIV gp120, 2F5 recognizes an epitope on HIV gp41. Results revealed that two murine monoclonal anti-E2 antibodies, IgG$_{2a}$M6 (M6) and IgG$_1$M11 (M11), neutralized HIV in a dose dependant manner, whereas isotype control antibodies and the other six murine monoclonal anti-E2 antibodies did not suppress HIV (Figure 5-31). For further evaluation, another neutralization assays on CEMx174$_{CCR5}$ cells using HIV$_{PP}$ bearing the envelope of CCR5- and CXCR4-tropic HIV, SIV, MLV or VSV, were performed. Comparable to HIV$_{WT}$ propagated on PBMC and CEMx174$_{CCR5}$, also HIV$_{PP}$ were inhibited by anti-E2 positive IgG fractions as well as by the anti-E2 antibodies M6 and M11. Again, the data confirmed a broad reactivity of M6 and M11 (IC$_{50}$ ranging from 0.03µg/ml to 0.08µg/ml). Noteworthy, not only HIV$_{gp120}$ enveloped HIV$_{PP}$ were inhibited by anti-E2 antibodies, but also HIV$_{PP}$ enveloped with SIV$_{gp130}$, MLV$_{gp80}$, and VSV$_G$. As expected, the HIV-neutralizing antibodies 2G12, 2F5, and F425B4e8 displayed a comparable potency for HIV$_{gp120}$ enveloped HIV$_{PP}$, but failed to neutralize HIV$_{PP}$ with homologous envelopes (Figure 5-32). Taken together, the data suggest

a)

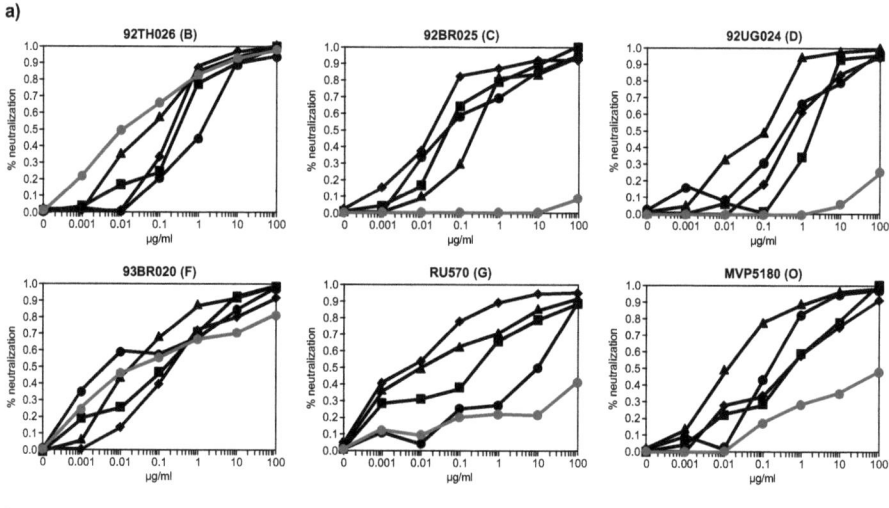

b)

| | 92TH026 | 92BR025 | 92UG024 | 93BR020 | RU570 | MVP5180 | JR-CSF | NL4-3 | YU-2 |
|---|---|---|---|---|---|---|---|---|---|
| | | | | | $IC_{50}$ [µg/ml] | | | | |
| | human polyclonal IgG fractions of anti-E2 positive (+) and anti-E2 negative (–) donors | | | | | | | | |
| 0105 (+) | 0.080 | 0.242 | 0.084 | 0.027 | 0.008 | 0.024 | 0.029 | 0.003 | 0.081 |
| 0818 (+) | 1.053 | 0.090 | 0.381 | 0.037 | 6.078 | 0.158 | 0.418 | 0.013 | 0.056 |
| 1001 (–) | >100 | >100 | >100 | >100 | >100 | >100 | >100 | >100 | >100 |
| 1404 (+) | 0.177 | 0.025 | 0.476 | 0.334 | 0.008 | 0.428 | 0.024 | 0.628 | 0.238 |
| 1619 (–) | >100 | >100 | >100 | >100 | >100 | >100 | >100 | >100 | >100 |
| 1910 (–) | >100 | >100 | >100 | >100 | >100 | >100 | >100 | >100 | >100 |
| 1918 (+) | 0.217 | 0.075 | 2.150 | 0.132 | 0.185 | 0.453 | 0.525 | 0.166 | 0.001 |
| 2511 (–) | >100 | >100 | >100 | >100 | >100 | >100 | >100 | >100 | >100 |
| | murine monoclonal anti-E2 antibodies | | | | | | | | |
| MAb M3 | >100 | >100 | >100 | >100 | >100 | >100 | >100 | >100 | >100 |
| MAb M5 | >100 | >100 | >100 | >100 | >100 | >100 | >100 | >100 | >100 |
| MAb M6 | 0.045 | 0.046 | 0.420 | 0.924 | 1.957 | 0.010 | 0.091 | 0.287 | 0.077 |
| MAb M11 | 0.095 | 0.155 | 0.036 | 0.089 | 1.510 | 0.040 | 0.111 | 0.842 | 0.148 |
| MAb M13 | >100 | >100 | >100 | >100 | >100 | >100 | >100 | >100 | >100 |
| MAb M17 | >100 | >100 | >100 | >100 | >100 | >100 | >100 | >100 | >100 |
| MAb M19 | >100 | >100 | >100 | >100 | >100 | >100 | >100 | >100 | >100 |
| MAb M30 | >100 | >100 | >100 | >100 | >100 | >100 | >100 | >100 | >100 |
| | human monoclonal anti-HIV antibodies | | | | | | | | |
| 2F5 | 0.020 | >100 | >100 | 0.064 | 3.127 | 68.025 | 3.802 | 0.921 | 47.011 |
| 2G12 | 0.022 | >100 | >100 | 0.068 | >100 | >100 | 0.401 | 3.273 | 65.469 |
| F425B4e8 | 0.009 | >100 | >100 | 0.301 | 0.948 | 56.902 | 0.054 | 26.184 | 38.688 |

Figure 5-31: Neutralization of HIV$_{WT}$ by anti-E2 antibodies. CCR5- (92TH026, 92BR025, RU570), CXCR4- (92UG024, JR-CSF, NL4-3, YU-2), and CCR5/CXCR4-tropic (93BR020, MVP5180) HIV isolates were incubated with anti-E2 or respective control antibodies. a) Curves show the concentrations required to achieve the designated levels of neutralization for the human polyclonal IgG preparations of anti-E2 antibodies positive blood donors 0105 (–▲–), 0818 (–●–), 1404 (–▼–), 1918 (–■–) and the monoclonal antibody 2G12 (–●–). Ongoing replication was observed and p24 antigen concentration was measured by ELISA to calculate percent neutralization in relation to mock. A representative experiment is shown. b) The table summarizes the concentrations (micrograms per milliliter) of polyclonal IgG derived from anti-E2 positive (0105, 0818, 1404, 1918) and negative (1001, 1619, 1910, 2511) blood donors, murine monoclonal anti-E2 antibodies (M3, M5, M6, M11, M13, M17, M19, M30), and human monoclonal HIV-neutralizing control antibodies (2F5, 2G12, F425B4e8) that inhibit the HIV p24 release of the respective primary or laboratory adapted HIV isolate by 50 percent (IC$_{50}$).

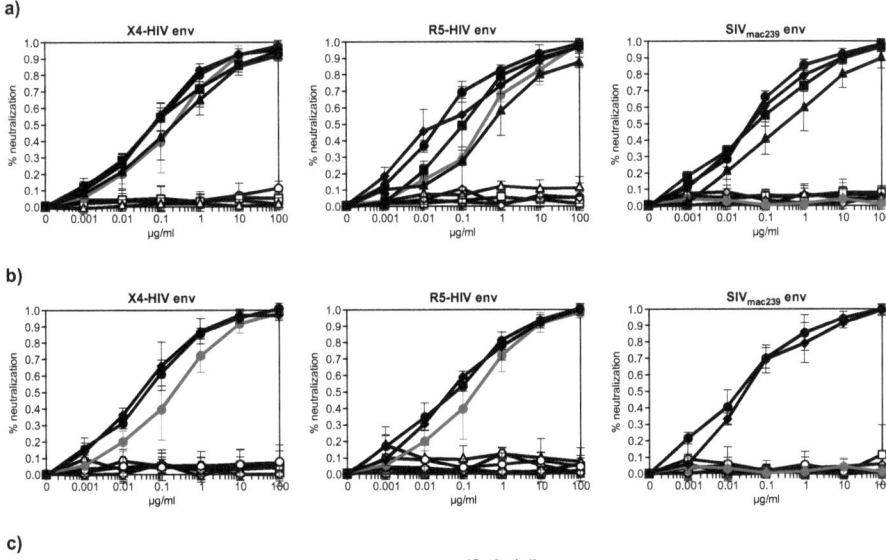

| | NL4-3 env | HxB2 env | ADA env | SIV$_{mac239}$ env | MLV env | VSV env |
|---|---|---|---|---|---|---|
| | \multicolumn{6}{l}{human polyclonal IgG fractions of anti-E2 positive (+) and anti-E2 negative (-) donors} | | | | | |
| 0105 (+) | 0.132 ± 0.034 | 0.415 ± 0.062 | 1.101 ± 0.118 | 0.388 ± 0.022 | 0.903 ± 0.006 | 0.737 ± 0.037 |
| 0818 (+) | 0.095 ± 0.021 | 0.062 ± 0.013 | 0.037 ± 0.005 | 0.060 ± 0.007 | 0.051 ± 0.006 | 0.145 ± 0.021 |
| 1001 (-) | >100 | >100 | >100 | >100 | >100 | >100 |
| 1404 (+) | 0.078 ± 0.003 | 0.063 ± 0.013 | 0.060 ± 0.017 | 0.066 ± 0.002 | 0.050 ± 0.011 | 0.084 ± 0.007 |
| 1619 (-) | >100 | >100 | >100 | >100 | >100 | >100 |
| 1910 (-) | >100 | >100 | >100 | >100 | >100 | >100 |
| 1918 (+) | 0.183 ± 0.019 | 0.058 ± 0.004 | 0.132 ± 0.033 | 0.076 ± 0.003 | 0.106 ± 0.016 | 0.380 ± 0.034 |
| 2511 (-) | >100 | >100 | >100 | >100 | >100 | >100 |
| | \multicolumn{6}{c}{murine monoclonal anti-E2 antibodies} | | | | | |
| M3 | >100 | >100 | >100 | >100 | >100 | >100 |
| M5 | >100 | >100 | >100 | >100 | >100 | >100 |
| M6 | 0.048 ± 0.004 | 0.064 ± 0.004 | 0.057 ± 0.006 | 0.033 ± 0.007 | 0.030 ± 0.003 | 0.351 ± 0.089 |
| M11 | 0.043 ± 0.019 | 0.036 ± 0.021 | 0.079 ± 0.006 | 0.064 ± 0.017 | 0.038 ± 0.008 | 0.150 ± 0.029 |
| M13 | >100 | >100 | >100 | >100 | >100 | >100 |
| M17 | >100 | >100 | >100 | >100 | >100 | >100 |
| M19 | >100 | >100 | >100 | >100 | >100 | >100 |
| M30 | >100 | >100 | >100 | >100 | >100 | >100 |
| | \multicolumn{6}{c}{human monoclonal anti-HIV antibodies} | | | | | |
| 2F5 | 0.475 ± 0.133 | 0.054 ± 0.013 | 0.061 ± 0.018 | >100 | >100 | >100 |
| 2G12 | 0.213 ± 0.021 | 0.083 ± 0.005 | 0.356 ± 0.039 | >100 | >100 | >100 |
| F425B4e8 | 12.853 ± 1.170 | 0.542 ± 0.078 | 0.885 ± 0.062 | >100 | >100 | >100 |

**Figure 5-32: Neutralization of HIV$_{PP}$ by anti-E2 antibodies.** HIV$_{PP}$ enveloped either with HIV$_{gp120}$, SIV$_{mac239}$, MLV or with VSV$_G$ were incubated with anti-E2 antibodies or human monoclonal HIV-neutralizing control antibodies and used to infect CEMx174$_{CCR5}$ cells. Luciferase activity in the cell lysates was measured 72 hours later. Data represent three independent experiments performed in duplicates. The curves show the mean concentrations of **a)** anti-E2 positive (0105 (-▲-), 0818 (-●-), 1404 (-◆-), 1918 (-■-) and negative IgG fractions (1001 (-○-), 1619 (-△-), 1910 (-◇-), 2511 (-□-)), of the **b)** murine monoclonal anti-E2 antibodies M3 (-○-), M5 (-△-), M6 (-●-), M11 (-◆-), M13 (-◇-), M17 (-□-), M19 (-◇-), M30 (-○-) as well as of the human monoclonal antibody 2G12 (-●-), required to achieve the designated levels of neutralization. **c)** The table summarizes the concentrations (micrograms per milliliter) of anti-E2 and human HIV-neutralizing control antibodies (2F5, 2G12, F425B4e8) that reduce the luciferase activity by 50 percent (IC$_{50}$).

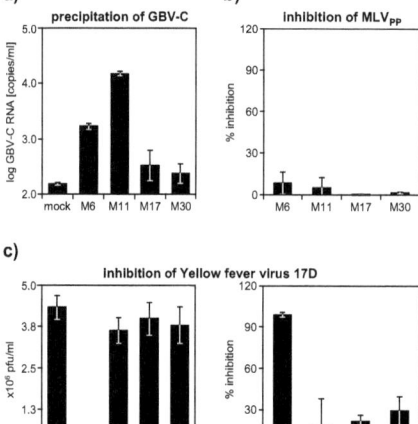
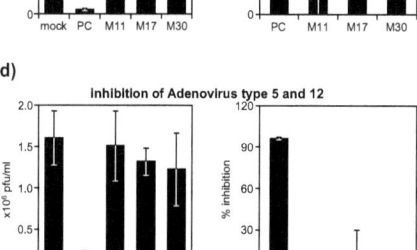

Figure 5-33: Neutralization ability of anti-E2 antibodies is restricted to HIV. a) GBV-C RNA positive serum was incubated with the anti-E2 antibodies M6, M11, M17, M30, and the respective isotype control (IC) antibodies (mock) and precipitated by Protein G covered Sepharose beads (Sigma-Aldrich, Deisenhofen). RNA of precipitated GBV-C was extracted and quantified by real-time RT-PCR. b) MLV$_{EGFP}$ pseudoparticles (MLV$_{PP}$) bearing CXCR4-tropic HIV$_{gp120}$ or VSV$_G$ envelopes were incubated with M6, M11, M17, M30, and respective IC antibodies prior TZM-bl cells were added. GFP fluorescence was measured by flow cytometry at day three post infection and inhibition was calculated in relation to mock. Average inhibition of three independent experiments performed in triplicates is shown. c) YFV$_{17D}$ was incubated with serum of a YFV$_{17D}$ immunized volunteer (PC), M11, M17, M30, and respective IC antibodies. Infectivity of YFV$_{17D}$ was analyzed in plaque assays on Vero-B4 cells (left) and in infection assays on PBMC. Replication capacity of YFV$_{17D}$ was quantified by real-time RT-PCR. Inhibition was calculated in relation to mock (right). Columns represent average values of three independent experiments performed in duplicates. d) Adenovirus (Ad) type 5 or 12 and recombinant Ad5$_{beta-Gal}$ were incubated with serum of a volunteer containing adenovirus-directed antibodies (PC), M11, M17, M30, and respective IC antibodies. Ad5 and Ad12 infectivity were analyzed in plaque assays on BHK$_{CAR}$ cells (left). Replication of Ad5$_{beta-Gal}$ was determined by the activity of beta-Galactosidase in cell lysates of infected Hela-CD4$^+$ cells. Inhibition was calculated in relation to mock. Columns represent average inhibition of at least three independent experiments performed in duplicates (right).

that anti-E2 antibodies target an epitope that is not present on HIV$_{gp120}$, but may be located within the lipid bilayer of mature HIV virions. Although all tested monoclonal anti-E2 antibodies are directed against the E2 surface protein of GBV-C, exclusively M6 and M11 were able to precipitate GBV-C particles from human sera suggesting a pronounced feature in virus particle recognition of M6 and M11. To evaluate, whether other viruses are recognized by HIV-neutralizing anti-E2 antibodies, the moloney murine leukemia virus (MLV, *Retroviridae*) the yellow fever virus (YFV), a GBV-C related member of the *Flaviviridae*, and the nonenveloped human Adenovirus type 5 and 12 (*Adenoviridae*) were tested for neutralization sensitivity. Noteworthy, none of these viruses could be efficiently neutralized by M6 and M11 indicating that the cross reactivity of anti-E2 antibodies is restricted to human retroviruses (Figure 5-33).

### 5.5.3. Mechanism of HIV Inhibition by anti-E2 Antibodies

To investigate the possibility that anti-E2 antibodies induced HIV suppression is mediated by induction of HIV-inhibitory chemokines, a neutralization assay on PBMC using the chemokine resistant HIV strain SF33 was performed. Comparable to 2G12, anti-E2 positive IgG preparations (0818, 1404) as well as M11 neutralized SF33 efficiently, whereas the anti-E2 antibodies M17 and M30 did not. In this assay, the control antibody 2F5 failed to neutralize SF33 (Figure 5-34a). Additionally, a single round of infection assay on TZM-bl cells in the presence of high anti-MIP1alpha, anti-MIP1beta, anti-RANTES, and anti-SDF concentrations

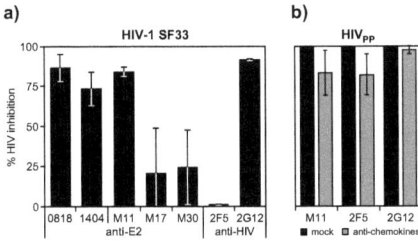
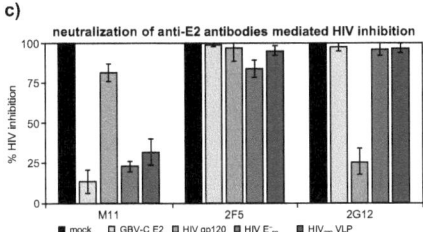

Figure 5-34: Neutralization of the anti-E2 antibodies mediated HIV-inhibitory effect. a) SF33 was incubated with anti-E2 (0818, 1404, M11, M17, M30) and control (2F5, 2G12) antibodies prior PBMC were added. Post infection, cells were washed and cultivated in RPMI$_{complete}$ supplemented with 1µg/ml of the respective antibody. HIV inhibition was calculated in relation to mock. b) HIV$_{gp120}$ enveloped HIV$_{PP}$ were incubated with M11, 2F5, 2G12, and isotype control (IC) antibodies. In the absence (mock) or presence of 200µg/ml anti-RANTES, 50µg/ml anti-MIP-1alpha, 100µg/ml anti-MIP-1beta as well as 100µg/ml anti-SDF-1, TZM-bl cells in DMEM$_{complete}$ with 15µg/ml DEAE-Dextran were added. Inhibition in the absence of anti-chemokine antibodies (M11: 67±12%, 2F5: 67±18%, 2G12 83±11%) was calculated by the luciferase activity at day three post infection, set to 100% and compared with the respective anti-chemokines treated approach. c) Antibodies were preincubated with 5ng E2, gp120, HIV E$^-$$_{PP}$, or HIV$_{Gag}$ VLP. Columns represent average inhibition of three independent experiments performed in duplicates. HIV neutralization capacity of pre-treated M11, 2F5, and 2G12 antibodies was compared with the untreated that was set to 100%.

was performed Hereby, the anti-chemokine antibody cocktail was not able to abolish the HIV-neutralization activity of M11 (Figure 5-34b). Therefore, chemokine induction by anti-E2 antibodies as the causative mechanism of anti-E2 antibody mediated HIV inhibition could be excluded. In addition, competition assays were performed to analyze the inhibitory activity of anti-E2 antibodies in more detail and to narrow down the nature of the binding target of HIV-neutralizing anti-E2 antibodies. For this purpose, M11, 2F5, and 2G12 were pre-incubated with GBV-C E2(340)-Fc, HIV gp120, HIV$_{PP}$ particles without incorporated gp120, and virus like particles (VLP) harvested from HIV$_{gag}$ expressing 293T cells. Whereas the HIV neutralization ability of 2F5 was not affected at all, neutralization by the anti-gp120 antibody 2G12 was exclusively suppressed by pre-incubation with recombinant gp120. As expected, preincubation with recombinant E2 protein decreased the neutralization activity of the anti-E2 antibody M11, whereas preincubation with HIV gp120 resulted only in a slight reduction of M11 mediated HIV neutralization. Noteworthy, the use of HIV$_{PP}$ without incorporated HIV envelope or gag-derived particles led also to a reduced neutralization ability of M11 suggesting that M11 binds

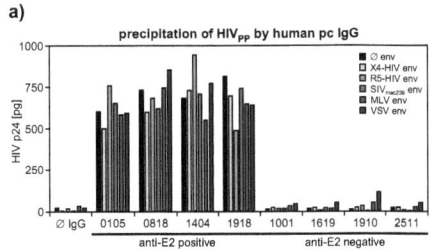
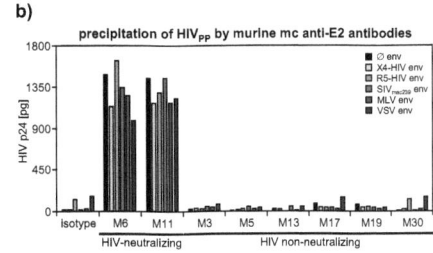

Figure 5-35: Immunoprecipitation of HIV$_{PP}$ by anti-E2 antibodies. Enveloped or non-enveloped HIV$_{PP}$ were incubated with purified IgG or anti-E2 antibodies, precipitated by Protein A or Protein G Sepharose beads and quantified by p24 ELISA. Pull down of HIV$_{PP}$ by a) human polyclonal anti-E2 positive (0105, 0818, 1404, 1918) and negative (1001, 1619, 1910, 2511) IgG preparations as well as anti-E2 positive sera without the IgG fraction (Ø) or b) by monoclonal murine anti-E2 antibodies (M3, M5, M6, M11, M13, M17, M19, M30) and respective isotype control antibodies (IC).

to HIV particles independent of the presence of gp120 (Figure 5-34c). Furthermore, immunoprecipitations of HIV particles were performed using enveloped and non-enveloped HIV$_{PP}$. IgG preparations derived from anti-E2 positive blood donors were able to bind and precipitate HIV$_{gp120}$ enveloped HIV$_{PP}$. In contrast, purified IgG from anti-E2 negative sera and anti-E2 positive sera without the IgG fraction did not. Accordingly, the anti-E2 antibodies M6 and M11 precipitated HIV$_{PP}$ as well, whereas the other six anti-E2 as well as control antibodies did not (Figure 5-35). Pull-down efficiency of HIV$_{PP}$ was not modulated by the presence of any viral envelope. Again, the data revealed that HIV-neutralizing anti-E2 antibodies recognize an epitope on the HIV surface that is not part of gp120, nor does the presence of this epitope depends on the incorporation of viral proteins. During the budding process, HIV acquires a lipid envelope derived from the plasma membrane of the host cell containing mainly cellular lipids and surface proteins as well as viral envelope proteins. Assuming that anti-E2 antibodies bind to HIV particles in a gp120/gp41-independent manner, the target of the HIV-neutralizing anti-E2 antibodies is expected to be located within the viral lipid bilayer as well as within the plasma membrane of HIV-producing cells. To investigate this assumption, cell binding capacity of M11, M17, and M30 was investigated by flow cytometry. Interestingly, a slight binding ability of M11 to native 293T cells could be observed that was greatly enhanced after fixation with paraformaldehyde (PFA) and even more after PFA-fixation and permeabilization with saponine. In contrast, no cell binding by the non-HIV-neutralizing antibodies M17 and M30 could be observed. The data imply the presence of a structure that is recognized by M11 and that is more accessible after fixation and/or permeabilization of the HIV producer cell. To test the impact of HIV protein expression on M11 cell binding, mock transfected 293T cells or

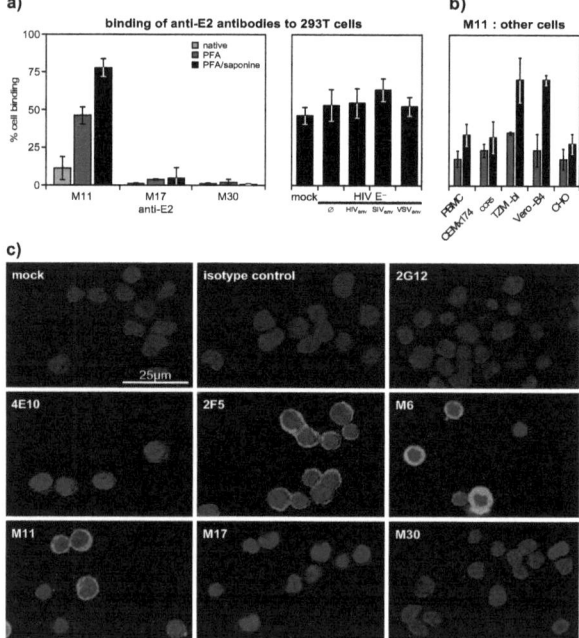

Figure 5-36: Cell binding by anti-E2 antibodies. a) Native, PFA, and PFA/saponine treated 293T cells were incubated with the anti-E2 antibodies M11, M17, M30 and respective isotype control (IC) antibodies (left). Mock transfected 293T cells and cells transfected with an envelope deleted proviral HIV genome (HIV E-) alone or together with plasmids coding the envelope of HIV, SIV, or VSV, were stained with M11 or the respective anti-IC antibody (right). Cell binding was analyzed by flow cytometry and %-binding was calculated in relation to mock. Columns show the average binding ability of three independent experiments. b) Binding affinity of M11 to PFA and PFA/saponine treated cells was quantified by flow cytometry in relation to mock. c) Immunofluorescence of PFA-fixed 293T cells, stained with anti-gp120 (2G12), anti-gp41 (4E10, 2F5), and anti-E2 (M6, M11, M17, M30) antibodies as well as the appropriate secondary antibodies (FITC, green). DAPI-staining of the cell nuclei was performed (blue).

293T cells transfected with an envelope deleted HIV proviral DNA construct alone, or in combination with plasmids coding for different viral glycoproteins. The data revealed that neither expression of an HIV genome nor co-expression of viral glycoproteins altered the presence of the anti-E2 antibody recognized structure on the cell surface of HIV producer cells. Additionally, the anti-E2 binding ability to PBMC, CEMx174$_{CCR5}$, TZM-bl, Vero-B4, and CHO cells were determined. Again, exclusively the HIV-neutralizing anti-E2 antibody M11 bound efficiently to all investigated cells and cell binding ability was enhanced after PFA-fixation and even more after PFA/saponine treatment. In order to illustrate the cell binding ability of the HIV-neutralizing antibodies M6 and M11, immunofluorescences of 293T cells were performed. Hereby, M6 and M11 clearly bound to PFA-treated 293T cells, whereas the isotype control as well as the non-HIV-neutralizing anti-E2 antibodies M17 and M30 did not. Interestingly, also the human anti-gp41 antibodies 2F5 and 4E10 bound to PFA treated cells, whereas no binding of the anti-gp120 antibody 2G12 could be observed (Figure 5-36). Since it was recently shown that antibodies directed against phospholipids are able to neutralize HIV in cell culture, the possibility, whether HIV-neutralizing anti-E2 antibodies would bind to lipids that are known to be present in the viral lipid bilayer[36], should be evaluated. For this purpose a membrane lipid array (Mobitec, Göttingen, Germany) was performed to test the binding ability of HIV-inhibitory as well as non-inhibitory murine monoclonal anti-E2 antibodies as well as of some human monoclonal HIV-neutralizing control antibodies. Indeed, M6 and M11 bound efficiently to phospholipids, whereas non-inhibitory anti-E2 antibodies did not. The HIV-neutralizing antibodies M6 and M11 detected phosphatidylinositol-4-phosphate (PI(4)P). M6 detected also other phosphatidylinositols, like PI(4,5)P$_2$ and PI(3,4,5)P$_3$. In contrast, M11 recognized furthermore cardiolipin that was also bound by the non-neutralizing anti-E2 antibodies M3 and M19. Therefore, it is unlikely that cardiolipin binding is involved in HIV neutralization by M6 and M11. Since it could

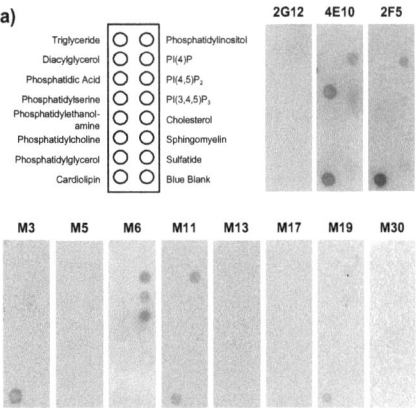

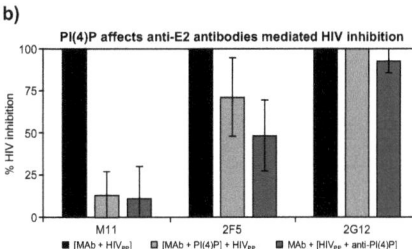

Figure 5-37: Binding of anti-E2 antibodies to phosphatidylinositols. a) Illustration of a membrane lipid strip. Stripes were incubated with 2F5, 2G12, and 4E10 as well as M3, M5, M6, M11, M13, M17, M19, and M30 prior bound antibodies were stained by HRP conjugated secondary antibodies and development by an ECL peroxidase substrate. b) HIV$_{PP}$ were incubated with M11, 2F5, and 2G12 and Neutralization capacity was determined on TZM-bl cells ([MAb + HIV$_{PP}$]). HIV inhibition was calculated in relation to mock, set to 100% and compared with the HIV inhibition of PI(4)P preincubated antibodies ([MAb + PI(4)P] + HIV$_{PP}$) and anti-PI(4)P IgM incubated HIV$_{PP}$ (MAb + [HIV$_{PP}$ + anti-PI(4)P]). HIV inhibition of PI(4)P-treated antibodies and anti-PI(4)P-treated virions was calculated in relation to the respective mock approach.

be shown that 2F5 and 4E10 are polyreactive and recognize a variety of lipids besides their epitope on gp41, reports from other laboratories could be confirmed[3,178,179,190]. Hereby, both anti-gp41 antibodies detected PI(4)P and cardiolipin, which is reported controversially for 2F5. In contrast, no lipid binding of the 2G12 antibody that is directed against carbohydrate structures as part of the HIV gp120 glycoprotein, could be observed (Figure 5-37a). Assuming that phosphatidylinositolphosphates are respective structures that were recognized by M6 and M11, competition assays on TZM-bl cells were performed. M11, 2F5, and 2G12 antibodies were preincubated with PI(4)P-covered agarose beads and subjected to neutralization assays. Additionally, HIV$_{PP}$ were incubated with anti-PI(4)P IgM prior HIV-neutralizing antibodies were added. Whereas the inhibitory capacity of 2G12 was not influenced at all, a slight reduction of the neutralization capability of the anti-gp41 antibody 2F5 was observed, which may be explained by the fact that phospholipids are part of the 2F5 epitope and that PI(4)P may play an important role in 2F5 membrane interactions. Remarkably, neutralization ability of the broad HIV-neutralizing anti-E2 antibody M11 was decreased in both settings suggesting an important role of PI(4)P in anti-E2 antibody mediated HIV suppression. Taken together, human anti-E2 positive IgG preparations as well as two murine monoclonal anti-E2 antibodies neutralized a broad range of HIV isolates by targeting PI(4)P within the viral membrane. For the first time, HIV-neutralizing antibodies could be elicited by a heterologous glycoprotein. In the future, these finding may lead to promising HIV vaccination strategies.

# 6. Discussion

Sexual activity and intravenous drug use are the most common routes of transmission among HIV infected patients. Since several pathogens, such as Hepatitis B and C virus (HBV, HCV), share similar transmission routes with HIV, it is not surprising that HIV infection is associated with such co-infections. In the course of HIV, coincident infections usually have been associated with higher viral loads and faster disease progression[64,123,126,284]. Co-infections with HCV induce higher morbidity and mortality rates in HIV positive patients[64,85,173,240]. Most notably, co-infections with the flavivirus GBV-C, also termed Hepatitis G virus, lead to delayed progression of HIV disease and improved survival of GBV-C/HIV co-infected individuals [287,308,317].

## 6.1. Effect of GB Virus C on HIV in Cell Culture

### 6.1.1. Replication Capacity of Clinical GB Virus C Isolates

To make a contribution to the clinical relevance of GBV-C co-infection on HIV suppression in humans, the current work investigates the impact of GBV-C on HIV under standardized cell culture conditions. For this purpose, a real-time RT-PCR was designed to quantify GBV-C virus load in different specimens and a bank of GBV-C positive sera was established. Since some reports provide evidence that GBV-C may be a lymphotropic virus[87,102,173], different B and T cell lines as well as PBMC and enriched CD4 and CD19 positive PBMC subsets were infected with clinical GBV-C isolates and viral replication was evaluated by real-time RT-PCR. Indeed, post infection of B and T cell lines as well as primary B and T lymphocytes the concentration of GBV-C RNA in cell lysates and culture supernatants increased over time indicating ongoing GBV-C replication. These results were supported by findings of Xiang *et al.* and George *et al.*, who demonstrated as well that GBV-C replicates predominantly in primary B and T lymphocytes[101,318]. Nevertheless, the overall virus production was transient and very low not exceeding $5 \times 10^4$ GBV-C genome equivalents per milliliter. Artificial effects due to mycoplasma or a cytopathic effect caused by GBV-C inoculation, which might explain limited GBV-C replication, could be excluded. However, since all of the investigated cell lines were established from patients with acute lymphoblastic leukemia, Burkitt or cutaneous T cell lymphoma, it is likely that modified karyotypes and/or polyploidy induces expression profiles of cellular receptors that are inconvenient for GBV-C infection. Furthermore, most of the cell lines are latently infected with other viruses, such as Epstein-Barr virus or Squirrel monkey retrovirus and secrete cytokines such as IL-2 and tumor necrosis factor alpha (TNF alpha), which may hamper GBV-C replication by viral interference or activation of cellular restriction factors, respectively. Since long-term propagation of GBV-C with up to $1 \times 10^8$ GBV-C genome equivalents per milliliter could be exclusively observed on human cord blood lymphocytes (CBL), it turned out that primary cells enable a better replication of clinical GBV-C isolates than human lymphoid cell lines. CBL contain multipotent hematopoietic progenitor cells at a higher frequency than PBMC and differ from adult PBMC in morphological and immunophenotypic cell features. An explanation for the increased replication capacity of GBV-C on CBL may be the relatively virgin status and greater number of immature T cells in CBL. In general, CBL have higher lymphocyte counts and larger subsets of CD4/CD8 double positive calls as well as larger subsets of helper/inducer and suppressor/cytotoxic T cells than PBMC[62]. Taken together, primary lymphocytes and notably CBL enable efficient replication of clinical GBV-C isolates. Even though, cells of different donors varied in terms of GBV-C susceptibility, variations in persistence and efficiency of GBV-C replication were mostly influence by viral determinants. Whereas some GBV-C isolates showed a strong and efficient replication capacity in cell culture, some isolates replicated very inefficiently on all tested cell donors. To monitor GBV-C replication by another approach, PBMC from GBV-C viremic individuals were isolated and cultivated. Again, GBV-C RNA was detectable in supernatants of most PBMC cultures for several weeks. The virus load ranged between almost undetectable and $1 \times 10^8$ GBV-C genome equivalents per milliliter. Thereby, replication efficiency neither did correlate with the GBV-C virus load in the serum of the blood donor, nor was they associated with the genotype of the GBV-C isolate or with the HIV status of the blood donor. It is likely that GBV-C isolates vary in their replication capacity on PBMC due to different cell tropisms. Studies of Fogeda *et al.* imply the existence of different GBV-C quasispecies in one infected individual depending of the source of the virions (PBMC, serum, liver)[87,102]. Since mutations within the envelope may affect viral replication, infectivity, and tropism[21,139,188,209], GBV-C isolates were sequenced and amino acid sequences of the envelope protein E2 were aligned. As supposed, different mutations within the E2 protein of clinical GBV-C isolates could be found, but in contrast to HCV, no hypervariable region was identified. Interestingly, GBV-C isolates replicating very inefficient in PBMC cultures, have accumulated several mutations that were not present in the E2 protein of high-replicative GBV-C isolates. Thereby, two mutations (E143K/H, T204A) were located in an area that is associated in the HCV E2 protein with CD81 binding and B cell epitopes of neutralizing antibodies[139,140]. To investigate the putative impact of these amino acid substitutions on protein structure and function, a theoretical three-dimensional model of the E2 protein was calculated using the I-TASSER server[237,322]. BepiPred, DiscoTope, and Seppa were used to predict B-cell epitopes[117,154,272]. These bioinformatical programs represent accurate and highly sensitive tools for specific structural and functional predictions using state-of-the-art algorithms. The computational methods suggest that E143K/H and T204A are either part of a linear B cell epitope or that they are closely related to a putative discontinuous B cell epitope. Substitutions of side chains affecting polarity and charge of the respective protein domain that may induce steric hindrance, could hamper the interplay of the GBV-C E2 protein with its cellular receptor. It could be shown for the HCV E2 protein that mutations located outside the known receptor binding sites can result in structural changes that lead to complete escape from neutralizing antibodies, while simultaneously compromising viral fitness by reducing binding to CD81[139,236,283]. Therefore, it is likely that E143K/H and T204A are responsible for the lower replication capacity of respective GBV-C isolates. Nevertheless, this assumption needs to be validated by further analysis including X-ray crystallography, NMR spectroscopy, and epitope mapping.

### 6.1.2. Inhibition of HIV Replication by Clinical GB Virus C Isolates

To investigate possible interference mechanisms of GBV-C and HIV in cell culture, PBMC were co-infected with GBV-C and HIV. Cell proliferation assays revealed that infection with clinical GBV-C isolates did not result in increased cell death or diminished metabolic activity. Nevertheless, the replication capacity of HIV was decreased on GBV-C infected cells. Thereby, clinical GBV-C isolates differed in their ability to inhibit HIV replication and three distinct phenotypes could be identified. The majority of GBV-C isolates impaired HIV and was classified as HIV-inhibitory. However, several GBV-C isolates inhibited HIV only within the first days post HIV infection or had no effect at all and were therefore classified as intermediate or HIV-non-inhibitory, respectively. Since human sera were used for GBV-C infection and most of the clinical GBV-C isolates were derived from HIV positive donors under antiretroviral therapy, sera from GBV-C negative, but HIV positive patients with comparable therapy served as negative controls. Furthermore, GBV-C virions were purified by sucrose density gradient centrifugation to exclude artificial effects caused by unknown drug levels or unrelated serum proteins. To avoid assay variations mediated by the genetic diversity of PBMC and multiple replication cycles of $HIV_{WT}$, single round of infection assays using $HIV_{PP}$ as well as the human T cell line CEMx174 were performed. As already observed in GBV-C/HIV co-infection experiments on PBMC, now, using the single cycle infection assay, again the same HIV-inhibitory phenotypes were observed. Noteworthy, $HIV_{gp120}$ enveloped $HIV_{PP}$ were impaired by HIV-inhibitory as well as intermediate GBV-C isolates, whereas $VSV_G$ enveloped $HIV_{PP}$ infecting target cells via endocytosis and independent of gp120/CD4 mediated membrane fusion, were exclusively inhibited by GBV-C isolates with $HIV_{WT}$-inhibitory phenotype. Taken together, the data imply that different HIV replication steps are affected by GBV-C. Whereas viral interference with HIV cell entry causes a short-term suppression of HIV replication, impairment of a further, post-entry HIV replication step is required for lasting and potent inhibition of HIV in cell culture. Interestingly, all HIV-inhibitory GBV-C isolates were isolated from GBV-C/HIV co-infected donors with long-term GBV-C viremia suggesting that co-existence for many years may be necessary to select for GBV-C strains with strong HIV-inhibitory abilities that affect early and late replication steps of HIV. Epidemiological data of Williams *et al.*, who could demonstrate that survival advantage of GBV-C/HIV co-infected patients was dependent on long-term persistence of GBV-C viremia, corroborate this assumption. Whereas the GBV-C status 12 to 18 months after HIV seroconversion was not predictive, the GBV-C infection five to six years after HIV seroconversion was significantly associated with prolonged survival among HIV positive patients[308]. Furthermore, the disability of some clinical GBV-C isolates to suppress HIV in cell culture, could not be explained by insufficient replication on PBMC, since no correlation between HIV-inhibitory phenotype and GBV-C replication capacity could be observed. Both, HIV-inhibitory and HIV-non-inhibitory GBV-C isolates displayed a low replication rate in cell culture.

### 6.1.3. Induction of beta-Chemokines by Clinical GB Virus C Isolates

Several reports revealed that infections with certain pathogens could transiently reduce the replication of HIV[12,223,238]. For example, influenza infection induces suppression of HIV replication by induction of type I interferon's[223]. Human herpesvirus type 6 inhibits CCR5-tropic strains of HIV by induction of RANTES and down regulation of CCR5[109]. To determine, whether GBV-C infection alters expression of HIV receptors on the cell surface resulting in decreased attachment and entry of HIV, expression of the HIV receptor CD4 and the HIV co-receptors CCR5 and CXCR4 was investigated by flow cytometry. Indeed, infection by HIV-inhibitory GBV-C isolates induced a significant decrease of CCR5 positive cells by CCR5 down regulation on the cell surface, whereas infection with HIV-non-inhibitory GBV-C isolates did not. Thereby, HIV-inhibitory GBV-C isolates stimulated the secretion of the beta-chemokines RANTES, MIP-1alpha, and MIP-1beta. Binding of these chemokines to CCR5 lead to reduced CCR5 expression and inhibition of CCR5-tropic HIV isolates. Furthermore, down regulation of CD4 and CXCR4 due to GBV-C infection was not observed, although a weak induction of SDF-1 could be measured. Thereby, the SDF-1 concentration in the cell culture supernatants was too low to be responsible for the observed inhibition of CXCR4-tropic HIV isolates. The data are in agreement with Xiang *et al.*, who showed that expression of mRNA for RANTES, MIP-1alpha, and MIP-1beta as well as secretion of the respective chemokine were higher in GBV-C-infected than in mock-infected cells[312]. Even though, induction of beta-chemokines and CCR5 down regulation by GBV-C would explain the observed inhibition of CCR5-tropic HIV isolates, this mechanism in unable to explain the inhibitory effect on CXCR4-tropic HIV stains and $VSV_G$ enveloped $HIV_{PP}$. Consequently, further mechanisms must be involved by that GBV-C interferes with HIV replication.

## 6.2. Interference of GB Virus C Proteins with HIV Replication

### 6.2.1. Generation of Human T Cell Lines Expressing GB Virus C Proteins

*Herpesvirus saimiri* (HVS) transforms human T cells and enables prolonged expression of foreign genes without decreasing HIV susceptibility. Thereby, the system allows long-term studies to investigate the impact of GBV-C protein expression on HIV replication[23,289,299]. Overlapping GBV-C gene cassettes were cloned in a HVS based gene-vector system and chimeric $HVS_{GBV-C}$ particles were produced. To generate human T cell lines expressing overlapping GBV-C gene cassettes cord blood lymphocytes (CBL) become infected with $HVS_{WT}$ and $HVS_{GBV-C}$. Although the viral genes StpC and Tip, which are required for T cell transformation, were present in the HVS genome, just a low transformation efficiency could be observed and was strongly depended of the CBL donor[193]. GBV-C protein expression increased over time and reached 90% at week 12 post transformation. Furthermore, cell surface expression of HIV relevant receptors was analyzed. Additionally, the impact of IL-2 treatment of CBL prior HVS infection was investigated in terms of the differentiation to CD4 or CD8 positive T cell lines of the initially CD4/CD8 double positive CBL. Whereas IL-2 stimulation had no effect on CCR5 and CXCR4 expression, it excited the differentiation to CD8 positive T cell lines. This is consistent with findings of Pacheco-Castro *et al.*[211] and may be explained by the biological function of IL-2 as a growth factor and its pivotal role in differentiation and homeostasis of effector T cell subsets including CD8 positive lymphocytes[19,161]. Additionally, expressed GBV-C proteins affected by CD4/CD8 differentiation as well. Whereas expression of the N-terminal part of the genome coding mainly for structural proteins, promoted CD8 differentiation, expression of nonstructural proteins supported maturation to CD4 positive cell lines. Thus, nonstructural GBV-C proteins may alter T cell activation that superposes IL-2 driven CD8 differentiation. Even though, it could not be excluded that T cell differentiation and/or receptor expression is affected by the interplay of GBV-C and HVS proteins.

### 6.2.2. Suppression of HIV Replication by Different GB Virus C Proteins

HIV infections of $HVS_{WT}$ and $HVS_{GBV-C}$ transformed T cell lines were performed. Thereby, HIV replication efficiency of GBV-C protein expressing cells was compared with that of $HVS_{WT}$ transformed cells. Surprisingly, expression of all three GBV-C gene cassettes hampered the replication of clinical HIV isolates suggesting that several GBV-C proteins exhibit anti-retroviral activity. Further single round of infection assays using HIV$_{PP}$ implied that different events in the HIV life cycle were affected. Whereas expression of the N-terminal GBV-C cassette inhibited exclusively the HIV-specific cell entry, impairment of VSV$_G$ enveloped HIV$_{PP}$ infecting target cells by a pH- and raft-dependent endocytic pathway, indicated that at least one nonstructural GBV-C protein may be involved in inhibition of HIV post-entry. To identify single GBV-C proteins that interfere with HIV in cell culture, each protein of the HIV-inhibitory GBV-C isolate AF121950 was cloned and transfected in CEMx174$_{CCR5}$ cells. HIV infection assays on transient transfected cells identified the HIV-inhibitory GBV-C proteins E2, NS3, and NS5A. In agreement with previous findings, expression of the E2 protein suppressed exclusively the gp120-dependent entry mechanism of HIV, whereas the nonstructural proteins NS3 and NS5A impaired later events during HIV replication. Taken together, these findings corroborate the assumption that GBV-C inhibits HIV replication by distinct mechanisms. Moreover, the data confirm the existence of different HIV-inhibitory phenotypes of clinical GBV-C isolates. Whereas intermediate GBV-C isolates impaired exclusively HIV-entry, potent HIV-inhibitory GBV-C isolates suppressed both, HIV-entry and HIV-entry independent HIV replication steps. Hereby, the ability to inhibit early HIV replication events, like binding and fusion, seems to be restricted to the GBV-C E2 protein. In contrast, the NS3 and NS5A protein impaired HIV replication independent of entry. Other studies support the finding that nonstructural GBV-C proteins are involved HIV suppression. Recently, it could be shown that the NS5A protein of GBV-C, HCV, Dengue virus, West Nile virus, and yellow fever virus is able to inhibit HIV replication by decreased steady-state CD4 mRNA levels and reduced cell surface CD4 expression[316]. Xiang *et al.* reported that the NS5A protein of GBV-C induces the release of SDF-1 and decreases surface expression of CXCR4. Deletion mapping of the NS5A protein identified an 85-aa region that mediates a strong inhibition of HIV replication in cell culture. Thereby, the serine at position 158 (S158) appears important for this effect[314,315] assuming that S158 is mutated within the NS5A protein of HIV-non-inhibitory GBV-C isolates. However, sequence analysis showed no substitution of the amino acids 149 to 238 of the NS5A protein of non-inhibitory GBV-C isolates. Although CD4 and CXCR4 down regulation might be responsible for the observed inhibition of HIV$_{WT}$ and HIV$_{gp120}$ enveloped HIV$_{PP}$, impairment of HIV$_{PP}$ with heterologous envelopes that evade the HIV-specific entry, could not be explained. Moreover, HIV inhibition by receptor down regulation seems to be a general effect of the NS5 protein of viruses of the *Flaviviridae*. In contrast, HIV inhibition by another, CD4-independent mechanism may be specific for the NS5A protein of HIV-inhibitory GBV-C isolates. Nevertheless, further experiments using several NS5A proteins derived from isolates with different HIV-inhibitory phenotypes are necessary. Independent of the NS5A protein, also the NS3 protease of GBV-C seems to mediate efficient impairment of HIV replication. Thereby, the inhibitory effect may be caused by the proteolytic ability of the NS3 protein. The NS3 protein of the related GBV-B cleaves the mitochondrial antiviral signaling protein (MAVS; also known as Cardif) and disrupt its function as a retinoic acid-inducible gene I adaptor and blocks thereby activation of the nuclear factor kappa B (NF-kappaB) and the interferon regulatory factor 3[47]. Since NF-kappaB has been shown to regulate the LTR-driven transcription of HIV[73,219,270], impairment of NF-kappaB mediated transcriptional activity could be responsible for the observed repression of HIV transcription in human T cell lines expressing the GBV-C NS3 protein.

### 6.2.3. Inhibition of HIV Entry by the GB Virus C E2 Protein

Taken into considerations that early events in the HIV life cycle have a tremendous relevance for HIV transmission, replication, and latency, therapeutics that prevent virus entry into new target cells and subsequently reduce the number of latent reservoirs for HIV, may have an advantage over existing therapeutic approaches targeting the viral enzymes reverse transcriptase, integrase, and protease. Therefore, the putative impact of the GBV-C envelope protein E2 on HIV inhibition was investigated in cell culture experiments. In accordance to other flaviviruses, it is believed that the GBV-C E2 protein belongs to class II glycoproteins and that it is incorporated in the viral membrane[16]. The assumption that the E2 protein is exposed on the virion surface is in agreement with the fact that anti-E2 antibodies are able to neutralize GBV-C infection[116,288]. In order to elucidate the role of the E2 glycoprotein on HIV suppression, a soluble GBV-C E2(340)-Fc fusion protein lacking the transmembrane domain, was cloned and eukaryotic expressed. Thereby, fusion to the human IgG$_1$ Fc fragment enabled easy and efficient purification via affinity chromatography, enhanced biologic activity, limited renal clearance as well as increased half-life as stated for many molecules, such as follicle-stimulating hormone and erythropoietin[26,74,125,255]. Moreover, soluble forms of the HCV E2 protein have been shown to be properly folded[186] and allowed identification of the cellular HCV receptors CD81 and scavenger receptor class B type I[221,247]. Therefore, recombinant E2(340)-Fc fusion proteins were a suitable tool to study E2/HIV interference. In contrast to the HCV E2 protein, which is heavily glycosylated, the GBV-C E2 protein has only three predicted glycosylation sites. PNGaseF digestion of the E2(340)-Fc fusion protein reduces the molecular weight by approximately 20kDa that is consistent with observations made for the full-length E2[278]. Truncated E2(340)-Fc proteins were expressed as homodimers mediated by the hinge region of the Fc fragment. Incubation of PBMC and human T cell lines with full-length E2 or truncated E2(340)-Fc proteins derived from GBV-C isolates with HIV-inhibitory or intermediate phenotype led to significant and dose-dependent suppression of HIV replication. In contrast, E2(340)-Fc proteins derived from HIV-non-inhibitory GBV-C isolates as well as the sole Fc fragment did not affect HIV. Using HIV$_{gp120}$ and VSV$_G$ enveloped HIV$_{PP}$, it could be shown that exclusively the HIV-specific cell entry was sensitive to E2-mediated inhibition. The half-maximal inhibitory concentration (IC$_{50}$) of HIV-inhibitory E2 proteins ranged between 5 and 7nM[130] and was comparable to those of other highly potent HIV-inhibitory proteins[20,196,275]. Cell toxicity as a reason for HIV inhibition could be excluded. Although previous sequence analysis suggested that the E2 amino acids E143 and T204 might be relevant for the HIV-inhibitory phenotype of clinical GBV-C isolates, linear 20mer peptides corresponding to the respective parenteral amino acid sequences, were unable to mediate HIV inhibition as observed for recombinant E2 proteins. Nevertheless, an impact could not be excluded, since these amino acids may be part of a three-dimensional structure that is causative for efficient inhibition of HIV-entry. Cellular entry by HIV is based on the interaction of the retroviral glycoproteins gp120 and gp41 with CD4 and CCR5 or CXCR4. To elucidate the mechanism of E2-mediated suppression of HIV entry, expression of HIV relevant cellular receptors after E2 stimulation was investigated. Recombinant E2 led to a significant reduction of CCR5 on the cell surface of PBMC, whereas expression of CXCR4 and CD4 was not affected. This is in agreement with Nattermann *et al.*, who observed down regulation of CCR5 upon stimulation with full-length E2[195]. Furthermore, this observation is in accordance with previous findings that infection of PBMC with clinical GBV-C isolates induces only a decreased expression of CCR5, whereas surface presentation of CXCR4 and CD4 was not influenced[131]. Comparable results were published by Xiang *et al.*, who observed the induction of alpha- and beta-chemokines[312]. However, stimulation with recombinant E2 induced just a moderate release of RANTES, MIP-1alpha, and MIP-1beta that cannot account for HIV inhibition, since E2 stimulation suppressed not only CCR5-tropic, but also CXCR4-tropic HIV. Therefore, it is likely that down regulation and chemokine induction presents side effects and not the major mechanism of E2-mediated HIV inhibition. Hence, the GBV-C E2 protein seems to be an HIV-entry inhibitor that interferes directly with attachment, CD4 binding, conformational changes of gp120 or membrane fusion. Since cell binding by E2 might block HIV receptor binding sites, E2 cell binding ability and expression pattern of selected surface receptors of several cell lines was combined. The data implied that CD3, CD4, CD8, CD19, CCR5, CXCR4, and CD81 were not necessary for E2 cell binding. Furthermore, the number of CCR5 positive cells was not decreased by a masking effect. Kaufman *et al.* corroborate the finding that CCR5 and CD81 are not the cellular binding partners for the GBV-C E2 protein[138] contradicting previous findings of Nattermann *et al.*[195]. Although preincubation of HIV target cells with recombinant E2 was sufficient to establish an HIV-inhibitory effect, it is likely that remaining E2 in the cell culture supernatant binds to structures on the surface of HIV particles thus inhibiting HIV cell binding and/or fusion and thereby, HIV replication. This assumption is supported by findings of Herrera *et al.*, who demonstrated recently that a peptide representing a region close to the E2 transmembrane domain, interacts with the gp41 fusion peptide of HIV[122]. Conformational changes of gp41 due to binding of the GBV-C E2 protein may block the triggering of the HIV cell fusion process and could be part of the underlying mechanism of E2-mediated inhibition of HIV entry. Even though, further experiments are necessary.

### 6.3. Impairment of HIV Infectivity by anti-E2 Antibodies

Inhibition of HIV replication by several GBV-C proteins, in particular inhibition of the gp120/CD4-dependent HIV entry by the GBV-C E2 protein, may be causal for the survival benefit of GBV-C/HIV co-infected patients. However, two epidemiological studies could also demonstrate that not only GBV-C/HIV co-infected individuals, but also those, who cleared GBV-C infection by the development of anti-E2 antibodies, display an increased survival in contrast to GBV-C negative HIV patients[287,308]. Therefore, the beneficial effect of GBV-C on HIV progression may be based upon a combination of direct viral interference mechanisms as well as induction of cross-neutralizing antibodies elicited by the GBV-C E2 protein. To analyze, if anti-E2 antibodies cross react with HIV particles, purified immunoglobulin G (IgG) fractions of several HIV and HCV antibodies and HBs antigen negative, but anti-E2 antibodies positive volunteers were tested in HIV neutralization assays. Indeed, anti-E2 positive IgG preparations neutralized HIV efficiently, whereas anti-E2 negative IgG preparations did not. Furthermore, two murine monoclonal anti-E2 antibodies, M6 and M11, could be identified that displayed the same cross-reactivity and ability to neutralize HIV. Human anti-E2 positive IgG fractions as well as the murine anti-E2 antibodies M6 and M11 displayed a broad activity against a variety of HIV isolates, comparably to the potent human monoclonal HIV-neutralizing antibodies 2G12, 2F5, and 4E10. Interestingly, M6 and M11 compete with each other, but whereas M11 recognizes a conformational epitope that is not well defined, M6 detects a linear epitope within the C-terminus of the GBV-C E2 protein that is involved in E2 cell binding[184,252]. This immunodominant antigenic site displays no significant homology with HIV or cellular proteins. Although the underlying mechanism is not completely understood and further experiments are necessary, initial data reveal that anti-E2 antibodies mediate HIV neutralization by binding to cellular structures on HIV virions. Thereby, HIV-neutralizing anti-E2 antibodies bound independent of the presence of the HIV glycoprotein gp120 to phosphatidylinositol-4-phosphate (PI(4)P) within the membrane of HIV particles. Nevertheless, it could not be exclude that PI(4)P are only part of the epitope and that viral glycoproteins or most likely, cellular proteins that are present within the retroviral bilayer may additionally be involved. The possibility that a further structure is recognized would explain, why anti-E2 antibodies do not neutralize other enveloped viruses like YFV or MLV. Especially in the light of the work of Chan et al. that could show that HIV as well as MLV virions are enriched in phophoinositides [44], the observed restriction to lentiviruses could not be explained. Since the viral lipid bilayer of HIV is achieved from the host cell during budding, the structure that is recognized by HIV-neutralizing anti-E2 antibodies should also be present on HIV host cells. Indeed, flow cytometry based cell binding assays and immunofluorescence could demonstrate that HIV-neutralizing anti-E2 antibodies bind to cellular membranes. However, cell binding capability was weak, but increased remarkably after PFA-fixation and even more after permeabilization. The data suggest that anti-E2 cross-reactive epitopes are normally not overexposed on the cell surface, because membrane proteins cover them or because they are predominantly located within the inner layer of plasma membranes. It has been described that PFA-fixation induces a decreased activity of $Ca^{2+}$ pumps disturbing the asymmetric distribution of phosphatidylserines within the lipid leaflets[310]. Since PI(4)P is predominantly located in endosomal membranes and the inner leaflet of the plasma membrane[70,250,298,321], PFA-fixation may lead to redistribution and exposure to the outer membrane. For other phosphatidylinositides, such as $PI(4,5)P_2$, an impact in membrane binding of $HIV_{Gag}$ due to myristoylation of the N-terminal matrix protein, has been implicated[37,51,204,239]. Myristoylation sites could also be found within the GBV-C E2 protein. Hereby, the myristoylation sites are in close proximity to the putative fusion peptide, the M6 epitope, and to the transmembrane domain and may be necessary to subject the E2 protein to cellular membranes and thereby to ensure the conjunction with cellular phospholipids. Recent work from Barrero-Villar et al. could show that phosphatidylinositides play an important role in early events of HIV replication. After gp120 binding, conversion of PI(4)P to $PI(4,5)P_2$ is enhanced in HIV permissive lymphocytes and noteworthy, prevention of PI(4)P phosphorylation leads to HIV entry inhibition[15]. Corroborating this finding, Brown et al. created a phospholipid-targeting antibody, WR304 that binds to PIP and thereby neutralizes HIV concluding that lipids themselves could serve as targets for HIV neutralization and may be the ultimate goal of reverse engineering vaccine immunogens[36,179]. Noteworthy, it was recently shown that broad-neutralizing anti-lipid antibodies increase secretion of CCR5-binding beta-chemokines[92,100,191,197,215]. Brown et al. observed that anti-PIP antibodies are able to neutralize HIV replication on PBMC as well, but failed in HIV-neutralizing assays on TZM-bl cells[36]. In contrast to the findings reported in this thesis, these antibodies bind to monocytes and not to HIV particles. Thereby, binding to HIV target cells triggers the release of MIP-1alpha and MIP-1beta, which might explain the observed inhibition of CCR5-tropic HIV strains. The lack of SDF-1 induction in this studies as well as the ability of HIV-neutralizing anti-E2 antibodies to inhibit HIV independent of the co-receptor tropism imply another mechanism for anti-E2 antibodies mediated HIV neutralization. Furthermore, contribution of chemokines by HIV-neutralizing anti-E2 antibodies could be excluded by neutralization of the chemokine-resistant HIV isolate SF33 and by efficient neutralization of HIV particles in the presence of high concentrations of anti-RANTES, anti-MIP-1alpha, anti-MIP-1beta, and anti-SDF-1 antibodies. The fact that HIV-neutralizing anti-E2 antibodies are cross-reactive and target phospholipids within the membrane of HIV virions is remarkable, since the human broad HIV-neutralizing monoclonal anti-gp41 antibodies 2F5 and 4E10 targets phospholipids, too. Until now, there have been a number of attempts to produce neutralizing antibodies targeting the 2F5 epitope with disappointing success[190]. It has been shown that 2F5 and 4E10 consist of an unusually long third complementary-determining region of the heavy chain (CDRH-3) that is attracted to anionic host-cell lipids[3]. Both antibodies target viral epitopes in the membrane-proximal ectodomain region (MPER) of HIV gp41 by a two-step process. The viral gp41 targets are only exposed and available for binding for a very short time and the antibodies owe their neutralization success to their attraction to host cell phospholipids that brings the antibodies in the right place waiting to pounce on their viral target when it appears[4]. For the 4E10 antibody, it is reported that this interaction leads to a conformational change of the membrane buried and immunoprotected MPER, which enables a stable interaction of the antibody with the MPER and leads to efficient HIV neutralization[273]. Interestingly, within the E2 protein, the linear M6 epitope is also very closely located to the transmembrane region and the proposed fusogenic sequence, which is able to form an obliquely inserted alpha-helix within membranes as already described for HIV gp41[180]. In contrast to the situation during the course of HIV infection, the appearance of anti-E2 antibodies is consistently accompanied with the clearance of GBV-C viremia assuming a very robust neutralization mechanism. If potent neutralization of GBV-C infection by anti-E2 antibodies depends on a similar MPER-membrane-involved mechanism that is observed for the potent, but rarely induced MPER-targeting antibodies 2F5 and 4E10, it may help to understand how antibody or antigen design can be optimized to achieve broad and potent neutralization. Taken together, antibodies elicited by the GBV-C E2 protein interact with phosphatidylinositol-4-phosphate. Although targeting phospholipids may carry the risk of autoimmunity[45], no enhanced risk to develop an autoimmune disease is reported for GBV-C anti-E2 positive individuals. Moreover, antibodies directed against phospholipids are able to neutralize HIV in cell culture. Therefore, interaction of cross-reactive anti-E2 antibodies with HIV virions may at least in part explain the survival benefit of GBV-C anti-E2 positive HIV patients. However, the mechanism of anti-E2 mediated HIV neutralization is currently not completely understood. In conclusion, increased survival of GBV-C/HIV co-infected patients seems to be the consequence of different, independent effects: direct viral interference and cross-reactive antibodies.

# 7. Methods

## 7.1. Escherichia coli

### 7.1.1. Preparation of Chemically Competent E. coli

An *E. coli* colony was transferred into 25ml of SOB medium and the starter culture was incubated for 8 hours at 37°C/200rpm. In the evening, three 1-liter flasks, each containing 500ml of SOB medium were inoculated with 1ml, 2ml, and 10ml of the starter culture and incubated overnight at 18°C/200rpm. $OD_{600}$ was monitored until one of the cultures reached an $OD_{600}$ of 0.45-0.55. This culture was chilled on ice and cells were harvested by 3600g for 5 minutes at 4°C. Supernatants were discarded and drops of remaining medium were removed by a vacuum aspirator. Cells were washed twice in 100ml of ice-cold Inoue transformation buffer and resuspended gently in 10ml of ice-cold Inoue transformation buffer supplemented with 750µl of DMSO. The bacterial suspension was mixed by swirling, placed in an ice-ethanol bath for 5 minutes, and 100µl aliquots were dispensed into chilled 1.5ml reaction tubes. Aliquots were immediately snap-frozen by immersing the tubes in liquid nitrogen and stored at -80°C.

### 7.1.2. Transformation of E. coli

A tube of competent *E. coli* was removed from the -80°C freezer and thawed by holding the tube in the palm of the hand. Just as the cells thawed, the tube was transferred on ice and chilled for 10 minutes. For difficult approaches and to improve the uptake of DNA, cells were transferred into a round bottom PP tube and treated with 1/100th volume of 100mM EDTA and incubated on ice for 5 minutes. In addition, 2/100th volume of 2.25M DTT and 2/100th volume of 1.22M beta-Mercaptoethanol were added and incubated for further 5 minutes on ice. DNA (1/5th volume of the ligation reaction or 10-50 pg of supercoiled plasmid DNA) were mixed with 1µl of 0.5M $MgCl_2$ and 1µl of 0.M $CaCl_2$ and added to the prepared bacterial cells in a volume not exceeding 10% of that of competent cells. Next, cells were incubated on ice for 30 minutes prior the tube was transferred for 30 seconds into a preheated 42°C water bath. Rapidly, the tube was chilled on ice and 900µl of pre-warmed $NZY^+$ medium were added and incubated for 1 hour in a 37°C water bath. Bacteria were collected by centrifugation (1800g, 5 minutes), gently resuspended in 100µl of fresh pre-warmed $NZY^+$ medium, and spread over the surface of an agar LM plate, which was incubated at room temperature until the liquid has been absorbed. The plate was inverted and incubated overnight at 37°C. This protocol has been used for *E. coli* DH5alpha and HB101. For the *E. coli* XL1-Blue strain, a modified protocol without the initial EDTA, DDT, and beta-Mercaptoethanol treatment was used. Purchased chemical competent *E. coli* were transformed according to manufactures protocol.

**Transformation Efficiency**

Transformation efficiency of each batch was calculated by transformation of 10pg pUC19 according to the protocol below and was determined to be ~$1 \times 10^8$ per µg DNA (Figure 7-1).

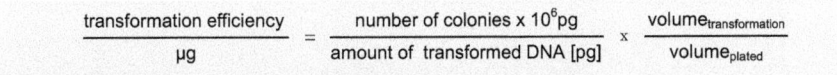

Figure 7-1: Calculation of the transformation efficiency.

**Long-term Storage of E. coli**
For long-term storage of transformed *E. coli*, a 2ml overnight culture was harvested, resuspended in fresh LB medium containing 50% glycerol, and stored at -80°C. To inoculate a fresh culture, a sterilized toothpick was scratched across the surface of the frozen stock and put into a flask with LB medium.

## 7.2. Preparation, Enzymatic Manipulation, and Analysis of DNA

### 7.2.1. Purification of DNA

**Preparation of Plasmid DNA**
Small-scale plasmid DNA was isolated by the NucleoSpin™ Plasmid QuickPure Kit (Macherey-Nagel, Düren). 2ml overnight culture were harvested, resuspended in 200µl resuspension buffer, and mixed gently with 200µl of lysis buffer by inverting the tube 5 times. To precipitate cell debris, 250µl of neutralization buffer were added, mixed thoroughly by inverting the tube, and centrifuged at 11000g for 5 minutes. Plasmid DNA containing supernatant was transferred to a NucleoSpin™ column and centrifuged at 11000g for 1 minute. The flow-through was discarded and silica membrane-bound DNA was covered with 450µl of wash buffer and centrifuged at 11000g for 3 minutes. The column was placed in a new 1.5ml reaction tube and dried by centrifugation at maximum speed for 1 minute prior 30µl of elution buffer were added and incubated for 1 minute. DNA was eluted by centrifugation at 11000g for 1 minute. High yields of plasmid DNA were isolated by anion-exchange chromatography (PureLink™ HiPure Plasmid Preparation kit, Invitrogen, Groningen). A 250 ml overnight bacterial culture was harvested, resuspended, and lysed according to manufactures protocol. All centrifugation steps were performed at 3500g. Cell debris was removed and clarified DNA containing supernatant was loaded on an equilibrated column, washed twice, and plasmid DNA was eluted into a 50ml reaction tube. An appropriate volume of isopropanol was added and DNA was precipitated at -80°C for at least 30 minutes and centrifugation for 1 hour at 4°C. The DNA pellet was air-dried, solved in $TE_{1:100}$ buffer and stored at -20°C.

**Preparation of Viral DNA**
Viral DNA from plasma, serum, and lymphocytes or cultured cells was isolated by the QIamp™ DNA Blood Mini Kit (Qiagen, Hilden) according to manufactures protocol.

**Resolution and Purification of DNA Fragments**
An agarose gel appropriate for the expected fragment size (Table 7-1) was prepared in 1x TAE buffer. Sample and size marker (GeneRuler™ 1kb DNA ladder mix, Fermentas, St. Leon-Rot) were loaded and separated at 100-150V prior the gel was stained in 1x TAE buffer containing 1µg/ml ethidium bromide and DNA was visualized upon illumination with UV light. Fragments were cut out and purified (QIAquick™ Gel Extraction Kit, Qiagen, Hilden).

| agarose gel [w/v] | fragment size [kb] | voltage [300mA] | time [minutes] |
|---|---|---|---|
| 2.0% | 0.1 – 1.0 | 150V | 90 |
| 1.5% | 0.5 – 2.0 | 150V | 80 |
| 1.0% | 1.5 – 7.0 | 120V | 50 |
| 0.5% | 5.0 – 25.0 | 100V | 60 |

Table 7-1: Conditions for agarose gel electrophoresis.

## Resolution and Purification of PCR Fragments

Quality of PCR fragments was analyzed by agarose gel electrophoresis. In the case of a single distinct DNA band, the PCR product was purified by the QIAquick™ PCR Purification Kit (Qiagen, Hilden). If multiple DNA fragments became visible, preparative gel electrophoresis was performed and the respective band was cut out and purified as described before.

### 7.2.2. Modification of DNA

#### Digestion of DNA with Restriction Endonucleases

Depending of number and size of expected restriction fragments, 0.1-5.0µg of DNA were mixed with the appropriate restriction endonuclease and incubated for 1 hour in 20µl of 1x restriction buffer at the recommended temperature. If possible, the restriction enzyme was inactivated at 80°C for 20 minutes or by adding EDTA to a final concentration of 12.5mM prior 5x gel loading buffer was added and the DNA fragments were analyzed by agarose gel electrophoresis. To cleave a given DNA with multi endonucleases that are active under the same restriction conditions, the enzymes were added together to the reaction mixture. If different reaction conditions are needed, a modified one- or two-step digest was performed. Reaction conditions reducing the activity of one of the enzymes by =50% were compensated by higher enzyme concentrations. Hereby, the total amount of glycerol did not exceed 1/10th of reaction volume. If the activity was reduced by more =50%, a two-step reaction was performed. Differ the restriction enzymes only in there reaction temperature, both enzymes were added and incubated first at the lower temperature prior temperature was increased. For double digestions at different salt concentrations, DNA was digested first in the low salt buffer prior salt concentration was increased and the other restriction endonuclease was added.

#### Fill-in Recessed 3'-Termini of Double-Stranded DNA

The Klenow Fragment of *E. coli* was used to fill-in recessed 3'-termini of double-stranded DNA. Therefore, 0.1-4µg of digested DNA in $H_2O_{dd}$ or 1x restriction buffer without EDTA were mixed with 1µl of a 1mM solution of each required dNTP, 0.5µl (5U) Klenow fragment, 10x Klenow fragment reaction buffer, and $H_2O_{dd}$ to a final volume of 20µl. The mixture was incubated for at least 10 minutes at 37°C prior inactivation at 75°C for 10 minutes.

#### Dephosphorylation

The release of 5'- and 3'-phosphate groups of up to 10pmol DNA termini (Figure 7-2) were catalyzed by adding 1µl (1U) Shrimp Alkaline Phosphatase (SAP), an appropriate volume of 10x SAP buffer, and $H_2O_{dd}$ to a final volume of 25-35µl. The mixture was incubated at 37°C for 1 hour and inactivated at 65°C for 15 minutes. Digestion with restriction endonucleases and dephosphorylation could be performed simultaneously.

$$\text{DNA ends [pmol]} = \frac{\text{amount of DNA [µg]} \times 10^6 \text{pg}}{\text{µg}} \times \frac{2 \times \text{pmol}}{\text{nucleotides [bp]} \times 660} \times \frac{\text{pmol}}{660 \times \text{bp}^{-1}}$$

Figure 7-2: Calculation of picomoles of DNA ends.

#### Ligation

A total amount of 200ng DNA in molar ratio of at least 1:3 of linear vector to insert DNA (Figure 7-3) were mixed with 1µl 30mM dATP, 0.5µl ligase, 1µl 10x ligation buffer, and $H_2O_{dd}$

to a total volume of 10µl. The reaction mixture was incubated at 22°C for 1 hour and used immediately for transformation of *E. coli*. Fore blunt-end ligation, reaction mixture was supplemented with 1µl of a 50% PEG solution.

$$\text{DNA [pmol]} = \frac{\text{amount of DNA [µg]} \times 10^6 \text{pg}}{\text{µg}} \times \frac{\text{pmol}}{\text{nucleotides [bp]} \times 660} \times \frac{\text{pmol}}{660 \times \text{bp}^{-1}}$$

Figure 7-3: Calculation of micrograms to picomoles of DNA.

### 7.2.3. Sequencing of DNA

To determine DNA sequences, a modified protocol of the enzymatic dideoxy method[241,242], combined with the BigDye™ Terminator v3.1 kit (Applied Biosystems, Darmstadt) was used. An appropriate amount of DNA (Table 7-2) was mixed with 3.5µl of 5x TM buffer, 1.5µl of 10µM primer, 1µl Big Dye™ ready reaction mix, and $H_2O_{dd}$ to a total volume of 20µl. Sequencing reaction was performed in a Mastercycler™ gradient (Eppendorf, Hamburg).

| template | Quantity | cycle sequencing conditions | | | |
|---|---|---|---|---|---|
| PCR product | | temperature control: | tube | | |
| 100 – 200bp | 5ng | temperature of the lid: | 98°C/wait | | |
| 200 – 500bp | 15ng | 1_initial Denaturation | 98°C | 1 min. | |
| 500 –1000bp | 30ng | 2_Denaturation | 98°C | 10 sec. | |
| >1000bp | 70ng | 3_Annealing | 50-60°C | 15 sec. | |
| plasmid DNA | 500ng | 4_Elongation | 60°C | 4 min. | 30x |
| Cosmid DNA | 1000ng | | 4°C | hold | |

Table 7-2: Amount template DNA and cycle condition for standard DNA sequencing.

## 7.3. Preparation and Analysis of RNA

### 7.3.1. In Vitro Transcription of RNA

RNA from the GBV-C clone AF121950 or respective deletion mutants were transcribed by the T7 MEGAscript™ kit (Applied Biosystems, Darmstadt). 1µg linearized plasmid or 1pmol PCR product containing the respective ORF and the T7 promoter were processed according to manufactures protocol. Templates were transcribed for 4-16 hours at 37°C. Remaining template DNA was removed by adding 1µl of DNase I and incubation at 37°C for 30 minutes.

**RNA Purification**

T7 transcribed RNA was diluted in PBS to a total volume of 200µl and purified by the High Pure RNA Isolation Kit (Roche Diagnostics, Mannheim) according to manufactures protocol. Purified RNA was used directly or stored at -80°C.

**RNA Agarose Gel Electrophoresis**

RNA was analyzed in comparison with a 0.24-9.5 kb RNA ladder (Invitrogen, Groningen) by denaturing agarose gel electrophoresis and ethidium bromide staining. 3µl sample or RNA ladder were diluted with 11µl sample buffer, mixed well with 1µl loading buffer, and denatured at 65°C for 5 minutes prior direct loading onto a 1% agarose gel prepared in ½ TAE buffer. Gel electrophoresis was performed at 80V for 100 minutes.

## 7.3.2. Isolation of Viral RNA

Viral RNA from plasma, serum, and cell culture supernatant was extracted using the QIAamp™ Viral RNA Mini Kit (Qiagen, Hilden). RNA of cultured cells was isolated by the RNeasy™ Mini Kit and the QIAshredder™ (Qiagen, Hilden). Cells were mixed with 350µl of RLT buffer. For further homogenization, the cell lysate was added to the upper reservoir of a QIAshredder™ spin column and centrifuged at maximum speed for 2 minutes. The column was discarded and the flow through was mixed with an equal volume of 70% ethanol. The sample including any precipitate that may have formed was transferred to an RNeasy™ spin column and centrifuged at 8000g for 30 seconds. 350µl of RW1 buffer were added and the column was washed by centrifugation at 8000g for 30 seconds. Genomic DNA contaminations were eliminated by an on-column DNase I digestion. A mixture of 10µl of DNase I stock solution and 70µl of RDD buffer was added directly to the RNeasy™ spin column membrane and incubated at room temperature for 15 minutes. To stop the reaction, 700µl of RW1 buffer were added and centrifuged at 8000g for 30 seconds. According to manufactures spin protocol for animal cells, the column was washed twice with RPE buffer and any possible carryover of RPE buffer or residual flow-through were eliminated by centrifugation at full speed for 1 minute. For RNA elution 30µl of nuclease-free water were added, incubated at room temperature for 1 minute prior a final centrifugation step at 8000g for 1 minute was performed.

## 7.3.3. Synthesis of c-DNA

To synthesize cDNA from viral RNA, the SuperScript™ III Reverse Transcriptase (Invitrogen, Groningen) was used. 5µl RNA, 1µl of 10µM gene-specific primer, 3µl of 10mM dNTP mix, and 3µl of nuclease-free H$_2$O were mixed, denatured at 95°C for 5 minutes, and chilled on ice for 5 minutes prior 4µl of 5x first strand buffer, 2µl of 0.1M DTT, 1µl of RNaseOUT™, and 1µl of SuperScript™ III RT were added, mixed, and incubated at 65°C for 50 minutes.

## 7.4. Mammalian Cell Culture

### 7.4.1. Isolation of Peripheral and Cord Blood Mononucleated Cells

**Density Gradient Centrifugation**

Peripheral blood mononucleated cells (PBMC) and cord blood lymphocytes (CBL) were isolated by Ficoll-Hypaque density (1.077g/ml) centrifugation. Blood was centrifuged at 500g for 10 minutes. The upper plasma layer was removed and stored at -20°C. The remaining buffy coat was mixed with an equal volume of room tempered PBS, layered on 10ml of room tempered Biocoll (Biochrom, Berlin), and centrifuged at 440g for 30 minutes without brake. The leukocytes containing interphase was collected and washed in RPMI. Cells were collected by centrifugation at 500g for 10 minutes, resuspended in RPMI$_{complete}$ to a final concentration of $2x10^6$ cells/ml, and cultivated at 37°C in a humidified incubator.

**Magnetic Cell Separation**

PBMC subpopulations were isolated by biomagnetic separation according to manufactures protocol. Untouched CD4 and CD8 positive T cells were enriched by negative selection using the Dynabeads™ technology (Invitrogen, Groningen), whereas CD19 positive B cells were separated by CD19 MicroBeads™ (Miltenyi Biotec, Bergisch Gladbach).

## 7.4.2. Cultivation of Primary Cells and Cell lines

Eukaryotic cells were cultivated in a humidified incubator (37°C, 7% $CO_2$, 80% $H_2O$). PBMC, CBL, as well as human derived T and B cell lines were cultivated in RPMI$_{complete}$ containing 50% Panserin™ 401, 10% FBS, 350µg/ml L-glutamine, 100µg/ml gentamycin. For stimulation of primary cells, growth medium was supplemented with 10U/ml of interleukin-2 (IL-2), 10µg/ml of phytohaemaglutinin (PHA) and/or 10µg/ml of LPS. Human embryonic kidney 293 cells containing the SV40 Large T-antigen (293T), Owl monkey kidney (OMK), Baby hamster kidney (BHK), Chinese hamster ovary (CHO), Vero-B4, Hela-CD4$^+$, and TZM-bl cells were cultivated in DMEM$_{complete}$.

## 7.4.3. Cell Proliferation Assay

The Cell Titer 96™ AQueous One Solution Cell Proliferation Assay (Promega, Mannheim) was used. 10µl of the MTS/PES solution were transferred into each well of a 96well plate containing target cells and the test substance in a final volume of 100µl growth medium. The microtiterplate was incubated for 4 hours in a humidified incubator, absorbance at 490nm was recorded, and cell viability was calculated in relation to mock treated cells.

## 7.4.4. Long-term Storage of Eukaryotic Cells

For long-term preservation in liquid nitrogen, cells were maintained in the actively growing state and culture medium was replaced 48 hours prior cells were harvested, transferred into a 15ml reaction tube, and chilled on ice. Cells were washed in ice cold PBS and resuspended to a concentration of $3 \times 10^6$ cells/ml in cryoprotective medium that was prepared according to the American Type Culture Collection (ATCC). Aliquots were added to prepared cryo tubes, sealed, and stored at -80°C for 24 hours prior transfer to liquid nitrogen. For cell recovery, a vial was removed from liquid nitrogen, thawed in warm water, and cells were washed in 10ml pre-warmed medium prior cultivation under standard growth conditions.

## 7.5. Transfection of DNA and RNA

### 7.5.1. Calcium Phosphate Transfection

Plasmid DNA was introduced to eukaryotic monolayer cell cultures by calcium phosphate precipitates that adhere to the cellular surface. The day prior transfection, exponentially growing 293T cells were seeded into tissue plates or cell culture flasks with a density of $2 \times 10^4$ cells/cm$^2$. Transfection was performed and 16 hours later the medium was removed and cells were washed twice with PBS, maintained in fresh growth medium, and incubated in a humidified incubator (37°C, 7% $CO_2$, 80% $H_2O$) unless otherwise specified.

**Transient Transfection using DNA Precipitates formed in HEPES**

For transient transfection approaches the HEPES standard protocol was used. Just prior transfection, the culture medium was changed. Highly pure DNA was diluted in $H_2O_{dd}$ and mixed with 2.5M $CaCl_2$. To prepare a fine calcium phosphate-DNA precipitate, 2x HeBS was pipetted into a sterile 50ml reaction tube, placed on a vortex mixer and the DNA/$CaCl_2$ solution was drop wise added, mixed for additional 20 seconds, and incubated for 15 minutes at room temperature prior the precipitate was layered directly onto the cells (Table 7-3).

|  | 293T cells | Medium | DNA$_{plasmid}$ | add H$_2$O$_{dd}$ | 2.5M CaCl$_2$ | 2x HeBS |
|---|---|---|---|---|---|---|
| 12-well plate | 8.7x10$^4$ | 1.2ml | 1.90µg | 90µl | 10µl | 100µl |
| 6-well plate | 2.2x10$^5$ | 3.0ml | 4.75µg | 225µl | 25µl | 250µl |
| 25cm$^2$ flask | 5.7x10$^5$ | 7.0ml | 12.50µg | 540µl | 60µl | 600µl |
| 75cm$^2$ flask | 1.7x10$^6$ | 21.0ml | 37.50µg | 1620µl | 180µl | 1800µl |

Table 7-3: Recipes for transfection mixtures prepared in HeBS.

## Stable Transfection using DNA Precipitates formed in BES

For stable transfection of fibroblast cell lines, an alternate BES-based method with higher transfection efficiency was used. The precipitate forms gradually in the cell culture medium under an atmosphere of 3% CO$_2$. To prepare an even, granular precipitate, 2x BBS and the DNA/CaCl$_2$ solution were mixed well and incubated for 5 minutes prior solution was added to the medium-covered cells (Table 7-4). Overnight incubation was performed in a humidified incubator with an atmosphere of 3% CO$_2$. To select stable transfected clones, culture medium was removed 24-72 hours later and cells were cultivated in fresh medium containing the respective selection marker.

|  | 293T cells | medium | DNA$_{plasmid}$ | add H$_2$O$_{dd}$ | 2.5M CaCl$_2$ | 2x BBS |
|---|---|---|---|---|---|---|
| 12-well plate | 8.7x10$^4$ | 1.2ml | 1.90µg | 40µl | 10µl | 50µl |
| 6-well plate | 2.2x10$^5$ | 2.4ml | 4.75µg | 80µl | 20µl | 100µl |
| 25cm$^2$ flask | 5.7x10$^5$ | 5.0ml | 12.50µg | 200µl | 50µl | 250µl |
| 75cm$^2$ flask | 1.7x10$^6$ | 15.0ml | 37.50µg | 600µl | 150µl | 750µl |

Table 7-4: Recipes for transfection mixtures prepared in BES.

## Production of HIV-derived Pseudoparticles

HIV-derived pseudoparticles (HIV$_{PP}$) bearing a CCR5- or CXCR4-tropic HIV$_{gp120}$ envelope or heterologous envelopes of the simian immunodeficiency virus (SIV$_{mac239}$), the amphotropic murine leukemia virus (A-MLV$_{gp130}$), or the vesicular stomatitis virus (VSV$_G$) were prepared by co-transfection of 293T cells with the envelope-defective proviral genome pNL4-3lucR-E- and envelope expressing plasmids in a molar ratio of 1:1 to 1:11 (Table 7-5). 293T cells were sowed into 75cm$^2$ cell culture flasks and when they reached 70% confluence, cells were maintained in 10ml of fresh medium. Plasmid and herring sperm DNA were mixed to a total amount of 40µg in a final volume of 400µl H$_2$O$_{dd}$, supplemented with 100µl of 2.5M CaCl$_2$, and mixed drop wise with 500µl of 2x BBS prior the solution was added to the cells. 24 hours later, the medium was replaced and when cells reached 100% confluence, supernatants were collected, filtered through a 0.22µm filter, and aliquots were stored at -80°C. HIV p24 antigen concentration and tissue culture infectious dose (TCID$_{50}$) were assessed.

|  | pNL4-3lucR-E- | pEnvelope |  | DNA$_{herring\ sperm}$ |
|---|---|---|---|---|
| Ø env | 10.0µg (1pmol) | 0.0µg |  | 30.0µg |
| NL4-3 env | 10.0µg (1pmol) | 10.6µg | (10pmol) | 19.4µg |
| HXB2 env | 10.0µg (1pmol) | 30.0µg | (10pmol) | – |
| ADA env | 10.0µg (1pmol) | 4.7µg | (3pmol) | 25.3µg |
| SIVmac239 env | 10.0µg (1pmol) | 7.7µg | (3pmol) | 22.3µg |
| A-MLV env | 10.0µg (1pmol) | 9.1µg | (3pmol) | 20.9µg |
| VSV env | 10.0µg (1pmol) | 17.1µg | (1pmol) | 12.9µg |

Table 7-5: Recipes for BES-based HIV$_{PP}$ production.

**Production of HIV-1 gag Particles**

HIV-1 gag virus like particles (VLP) were produced by transfection of 293T cells with the gag expression vector p96ZM651gag-opt from Drs. Yingying Li, Feng Gao, and Beatrice H. Hahn, obtained through the AIDS Research and Reference Reagent Program.

**Production of MLV derived Pseudoparticles**

MLV derived pseudoparticles were prepared by co-transfection of 293T cells with an envelope-defective proviral A-MLV genome and HIV-1$_{HxB2}$ or VSV$_G$ envelope expression plasmids in a molar ration of 1:11 and 1:2, respectively. Additionally, TCID$_{50}$ was assessed.

### 7.5.2. Electroporation

**RNA Transfection of PBMC**

PBMC were isolated and washed in PBS. $5 \times 10^6$ cells were resuspended in 100µl of the Human T cell Nucleofector™ solution, mixed with 5µg RNA in maximum 5µl H$_2$O$_{dd}$ and transferred air bubble free into a cuvette, placed into the Nucleofector™, and shocked using the program U14. When the program has finished, cells were resuspended in 500µl pre-warmed RPMI$_{complete}$, transferred into a 12-well plate, and incubated at 37°C in humidified incubator. Six hours post transfection the medium was replaced with RPMI$_{complete}$.

**DNA Transfection of CEMx174 Cells**

Exponentially growing CEMx174 and CEMx174$_{CCR5}$ cells were harvested, washed in PBS, and resuspended in Opti-MEM™ I with a density of $1 \times 10^7$ cells/ml. 10µg of DNA were diluted in 100µl Opti-MEM™, mixed with 100µl cell suspension, transferred air bubble free into a cuvette (gap width 2mm), placed in the Nucleofector™, shocked once using the program A30, and incubated for 5 minutes prior cells were transferred into 25cm$^2$ cell culture flasks with 5ml pre-warmed RPMI$_{complete}$. For stable transfection, cells were incubated for about two generations and then transferred to medium containing the appropriate selection marker.

### 7.5.3. Selection of Eukaryotic Cells

To determine the minimum required concentration, cells were incubated with various levels of the respective selection marker (Table 7-6). Every 3 days, cells were fed with the appropriate selective medium and examined for viable cells 2 weeks later.

| drug | tested range | 293T cells | CEMx174 |
| --- | --- | --- | --- |
| G418 | 100 – 1000µg/ml | 500µg/ml | 200µg/ml |
| Hygromycin-B | 10 – 500µg/ml | 100µg/ml | 200µg/ml |
| Puromycin | | – | 2µg/ml |

Table 7-6: Selection conditions for 293T and CEMx174$_{CCR5}$ cells.

## 7.6. Expression, Purification, and Analysis of Proteins

### 7.6.1. Protein Expression in Eukaryotic Cells

DNA was introduced into 293T and CEMx174$_{CCR5}$ cells by calcium phosphate transfection or electroporation. Expression and function analysis were performed 48-72 hours later. Stable cell lines were established by eukaryotic selection. Single cell clones were isolated by FACS.

### 7.6.2. Detection of Proteins

**Dot Blot**

A PVDF membrane was equilibrated in methanol and soaked in $H_2O_{dd}$. Per dot 20µl of cell lysate or 1µg of purified protein were spotted and were allowed to dry. The membrane was incubated in PBS/0.05% Tween-20/5% non-fat dried milk, washed 3 times with PBS/0.05% Tween-20 and was subjected to Western Blot analysis.

**Denaturing Gel Electrophoresis**

To separate proteins mixtures of cells or column fractions and to verify homogeneity of protein samples, one-dimensional, discontinuous SDS gel electrophoresis according to the standard method of Laemmli[153] was performed. According to manufactures instructions, the electrophoresis apparatus Mini Protean II (Bio-Rad, Munich) was used. To prepare the separating gel solution acrylamide and bisacrylamide were mixed in a ratio of 37.5 to 1 prior 1.5M Tris-HCl (pH 8.8), 10% SDS, and $H_2O_{dd}$ were added. Gel polymerization was initiated by addition of ammonium persulfate (APS, Merck, Darmstadt) and TEMED (Carl Roth, Karlsruhe). The staging gel was prepared in a comparable manner (Table 7-7). The gel cassette sandwich was placed into the electrode assembly and slid into the clamping frame. Finally, the inner chamber was lowered into the tank and inner as well as outer chamber was filled with 1x SDS electrophoresis buffer. To run the gel, sample pockets were rinsed with 1x SDS electrophoresis buffer and up to 20µl sample were mixed with 5x SDS sample buffer and heated 10 minutes at 95°C. 10-25µg of total protein or complex protein mixtures and 0.5-5µg of single proteins were loaded together with a molecular weight marker (PageRuler prestained Protein Ladder, Fermentas, St. Leon-Rot). Empty wells were filled with SDS sample buffer. Electrophoresis was performed for 90 minutes at 120V, 30mA until the bromphenol blue tracking dye reached the bottom of the separating gel. Electrophoresis buffer was discarded. The gel was washed once in PBS and stained with Coomassie blue. Alternate, the gel was blotted onto a PVDF membrane for subsequent staining.

| Stock solution | final acrylamide conc. separating gel | | | final acrylamide conc. stacking gel | |
|---|---|---|---|---|---|
| | 5% (60 – 200kDa) | 10% (20 – 90kDa) | 15% (10 – 50kDa) | 3% | 5% |
| 30% acrylamide | 1950 µl | 3900 µl | 5850 µl | 488 µl | 813 µl |
| 2% bisacrylamide | 780 µl | 1560 µl | 2340 µl | 195 µl | 325 µl |
| 1.5M Tris-HCl (pH 8.8) | 3000 µl | 3000 µl | 3000 µl | — | — |
| 0.5M Tris-HCl (pH 6.8) | — | — | — | 1200 µl | 1200 µl |
| 10% SDS | 120 µl | 120 µl | 120 µl | 50 µl | 50 µl |
| $H_2O_{dd}$ | 6018 µl | 3288 µl | 558 µl | 3007 µl | 2552 µl |
| 10% APS | 120 µl | 120 µl | 120 µl | 50 µl | 50 µl |
| TEMED | 12 µl | 12 µl | 12 µl | 10 µl | 10 µl |

Table 7-7: Recipes for denaturing polyacrylamide separating and stacking gels.

**Nondenaturing Gel Electrophoresis**

Under continuous conditions using the same buffer for gel preparation and electrophoresis, proteins could be separated by the pH value. Depending of the gel buffer, pH ranges from 3.7 to 10.6 and could be extended to pH 2.0 by the use of an unadjusted acetic acid gel buffer (Figure 7-4). For efficient polymerization at acid pH, the buffer was supplemented with 1/10th

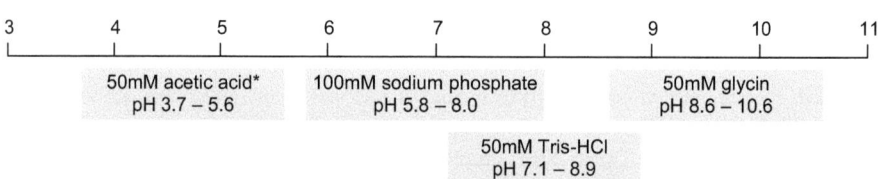
Figure 7-4: pH range of different electrophoresis buffers.

volume of fresh made sodium sulphite. Acrylamide solutions were prepared comparable to denaturing gels, but in the absence of denaturants such as detergents and urea (Table 7-7). Any charged material was removed by a pre-run at 300V for 30 minutes. Electrophoresis buffer was replaced and per lane up to 100µg of total protein solubilized in 5% sucrose were loaded. Isoforms and multimeric proteins were detected by discontinuous gel electrophoresis under native conditions. Samples were assayed by a minimum of 4 separating gels with different acrylamide concentrations, which were prepared without SDS and reducing agents as described before (Table 7-7). Samples were diluted with an equal volume of 2x Tris/glycerol sample buffer and electrophoresis was conducted under standard conditions using a Tris/glycine electrophoresis buffer. Separated proteins were fixed, stained, and relative mobility's were estimated. Therefore, a molecular weight curve was constructed by plotting the relative mobility against %T (%w/v of acrylamide/bisacrylamide).

**Western Blot Analysis**

Hydrophobic PVDF membranes were immersed in methanol prior gel, membrane, and filter papers were equilibrated in transfer buffer. Large proteins (>100kDa) were transferred by wet blotting. The transfer sandwich was assembled and air bubbles were removed by rolling a test tube over the surface prior the cassette was transferred to the blot module and placed together with the frozen cooling unit in the transfer tank. Transfer was performed at 100V and 350mA for 1 hour. Small proteins were transferred by semidry blotting. The complete transfer stack was placed on the anode of the blot apparatus, air bubbles were rolled out, and the top electrode was placed onto the transfer sandwich. Transfer was performed at 15V and 80mA for 90 minutes and verified by Ponceau S staining. The Membrane was washed in PBS/0.05% Tween-20 and blocked for at least 2 hours in PBS/0.05% Tween-20/5% non-fat dried milk. The respective antibody was diluted in PBS/5% non-fat dried milk and incubated for 60-90 minutes at room temperature prior the blot was washed and exposed for 1 hour to an horseradish peroxidase (HRP) conjugated antibody directed against the detection antibody. The membrane was washed again, equilibrated in 50mM Tris-HCl (pH 8.6), transferred to the visualization solution (prepared from 5ml of ECL solution A, 50µl of ECL solution B, and 2.5µl of 30% $H_2O_2$,), and analyzed immediately by a CCD-acquisition system.

**Stripping and Reuse of Membranes**

PVDF membranes were incubated in 50mM Tris-HCl (pH 7)/2% SDS/50mM DTT at 70°C for 30 minutes. For reprobing, the membranes were processed as described before.

### 7.6.3. Determination of Protein Concentrations

Total protein as well as purified recombinant proteins was quantified by Roti™ Nanoquant (Carl Roth, Karlsruhe) according to manufactures protocol.

### 7.6.4. Purification of Proteins by Affinity Chromatography

**Enrichment of 6x His-tagged Proteins by Metal-Affinity Chromatography**

Histidine tagged proteins were enriched by metal-affinity chromatography using Ni-NTA beads (Qiagen, Hilden). 100μl of the 50% Ni-NTA slurry were washed PBS, centrifuged at 5000g for 5 minutes, resuspended in 1ml of the respective sample, and incubated overnight at 4°C in an orbital shaker to kept beads in suspension. Ni-NTA bound proteins were washed twice in ice-cold PBS prior beads were mixed with 20μl 1x SDS sample buffer, incubated at 95°C for 10 minutes, and analyzed by SDS-PAGE.

**Purification of c-myc/His-Fc Fusion Proteins by Protein A Affinity Chromatography**

Fc fusion proteins as well as the sole Fc fragment were purified by HiTrap rProtein A columns using the ÄKTAexplorer™ system (GE Healthcare, Munich). Medium of 80% confluent 293T cells stable expressing the respective protein, was replaced with fresh DMEM$_{complete}$ (5% FBS) 48 hours prior cell culture supernatants were collected, treated with 0.25mM EGTA, adjusted to pH 7, and filtered through a 0.22μm filter. The column was washed with 10 column volumes (cv) H$_2$O$_{dd}$ and equilibrated with 10cv PBS (pH 7) prior supernatant was applied with a flow rate of 1ml per minute. Unbound material has been washed out by 10cv PBS (pH 7) and target protein was eluted in 0.1M citric acid by a linear decrease from pH 5 to pH 3. Fractions were collected and neutralized immediately by 1M Tris-HCl (pH 9). Alternatively, c-myc/His-Fc fusion proteins were purified by His MultiTrap HP columns. The column was equilibrated with 20mM sodium phosphate/500mM NaCl/20mM imidazole/0.5mM TCEP/1% TritonX-100 (pH 7.4). Cell culture supernatant containing recombinant Histidine fusion proteins were applied with a flow rate of 0.5ml per minute. Unbound material has been washed out by 10cv 20mM sodium phosphate/500mM NaCl/20mM imidazole/0.5mM TCEP/0.03% DDM/1% TritonX-100 (pH 7.4). Protein was eluted by 20mM sodium phosphate/500mM NaCl/500mM imidazole/0.5mM TCEP/0.03% DDM/1% TritonX-100 (pH 7.4). Finally, the column was washed (10cv H$_2$O$_{dd}$), reequilibrated (10cv 10x binding buffer, 10cv H$_2$O$_{dd}$), soaked in 20% ethanol (10cv), and stored at 4°C. Precipitated or denatured substances were removed by 5cv of 5M guanidine hydrochloride, hydrophobically bound substances by 5cv of 70% ethanol or PBS/1% TritonX-100 (pH 7). Immediately, the column was washed with 10cv PBS (pH 7) and 10cv H$_2$O$_{dd}$. The column was recharged by loading 2.5 ml of 0.1 M NiSO4 in distilled water.

**Purification of Human IgG by Protein A/G Affinity Chromatography**

Human IgG was purified and separated by multi step affinity chromatography using HiTrap rProtein A and Protein G columns. Serum or plasma was collected, inactivated at 56°C for 1 hour, and centrifuged at 3500g for 15 minutes. Supernatant was carefully removed, diluted with four volumes of PBS, supplemented with 1mM EDTA, adjusted to pH 7, filtered through a 0.22μm filter, and degassed. The whole IgG fraction was isolated by Protein G. Due to different binding affinities of the four IgG subclasses to Protein A and G, next IgG$_1$, IgG$_2$, and IgG$_4$ were isolated via a HiTrap rProtein A FF column, whereas IgG$_3$ remained in the flow through. Columns were washed with 10cv H$_2$O$_{dd}$ and equilibrated with 10cv 20mM sodium phosphate buffer (pH 7) prior sample was loaded with a flow rate of 0.5ml per minute. To wash out unbound sample, the column was rinsed with 10cv 20mM sodium phosphate buffer. Protein A bound immunoglobulins were eluted in 0.1M glycine-HCl by a pH step gradient of pH 6 to pH 2. Fractions were collected and neutralized immediately by 1M Tris-HCl (pH 9).

## 7.6.5. Deglycosilation of Proteins

N-linked glycans were enzymatically removed by Peptide-N-glycosidase F (PNGase F, New England Biolabs, Frankfurt/M.) that cleaves between the innermost GlcNAc and asparagine residues of high mannose, hybrid, and complex oligosaccharides from N-linked glycoproteins. 18µl of protein were mixed with 2µl of 10x glycoprotein denaturing buffer and heated at 98°C for 10 minutes prior 3µl of 10x G7 buffer, 3µl of 10% NP-40, 3µl of $H_2O_{dd}$, and 1µl of PNGase F were added and incubated for 2 hour at 37°C.

## 7.7. Incubation Assays

### 7.7.1. Incubation of Human T Cells with GBV-C E2-Fc Fusion Proteins

PBMC were harvested, washed in RPMI$_{complete}$ and resuspended in RPMI$_{complete}$ to a final concentration of $5x10^6$ cells/ml. To block Fc gamma receptors on the cell surface, 100µl cell suspension were mixed with 1µg of human IgG and incubated for 1 hour in a humidified incubator at 37°C. Cells were washed in 50ml PBSo and centrifuged at 500g for 10 minutes. Supernatant was discarded and cells were resuspended in PBSo to a final concentration of $4x10^7$ cells/ml. For each approach $6x10^6$ PBMC were placed in 4ml reaction tubes and mixed with different amounts of recombinant E2-Fc fusion protein and the sole Fc fragment, respectively. Incubation was performed under gently agitation in a total volume of 200µl for 45 minutes at 4°C. Again, the cells were washed, harvested, and resuspended in RPMI$_{complete}$ supplemented with IL-2 and PHA to a final concentration of $5x10^6$ PBMC/ml. For HIV$_{PP}$ infection, 100µl cell suspension were added per well of a 96well plate. For HIV$_{WT}$ infection or to produce supernatants of E2-Fc or sole Fc fragment stimulated PBMC, cells were diluted to a final concentration of $2x10^6$/ml, placed in a 12well plate, and incubated for at least 24 hours.

### 7.7.2. Incubation of HIV-1 Pseudoparticles with anti-E2 Antibodies

HIV$_{PP}$ were diluted in RPMI$_{complete}$ to a final volume of 50µl/well and transferred into a 96well plate. Triplicates were supplemented either with 50µl human sera, purified IgG with or without anti-E2 antibodies, or murine monoclonal anti-E2 antibodies. Incubation was performed in a humidified incubator at 37°C for 1 hour prior $5x10^5$ CEMx174$_{CCR5}$ in 100µl RPMI$_{complete}$ or $1x10^5$ TZM-bl cells in 100µl DMEM$_{complete}$ supplemented with 30µg/ml DEAE-Dextran were added. Three days later cells were harvested and screened for HIV infection. For measurement of expressed luciferase activity, 50µl lysis buffer were added per well, and cell lysates were transferred into a white microtiter plate. The luminescent reaction was triggered by injection of 100µl luciferase reaction buffer and the emitted light is recorded with a delay of 2.05 seconds.

### 7.7.3. IC$_{50}$

CEMx174$_{CCR5}$ or TZM-bl cells were incubated in quadruplicates with different amounts of recombinant GBV-C E2 protein or anti-E2 antibodies. HIV infection was performed as described. Wells are scored positive or negative for HIV infection by measuring expressed p24 antigen in the culture supernatants after seven days or by measuring luciferase activity in the cell lysates after three days. The average inhibition of each protein or antibody dilution was determined and the 50% inhibitory concentration (IC$_{50}$) was estimated.

## 7.8. Infection Assays
### 7.8.1. GBV-C Infection of Primary Cells and Cell Lines
PBMC and CBL were stimulated for at least 2 days with IL2 and PHA or LPS. Cell lines were split 24-48 hours prior GBV-C infection. $2 \times 10^6$ primary or $2 \times 10^5$ immortalized cells were inoculated for 4 hours at 37°C with GBV-C positive serum or plasma corresponding to $4 \times 10^6$ genome equivalents. Infection volume was adjusted with RPMI$_{complete}$ to 500µl. Post infection, cells were washed in PBS, maintained in RPMI$_{complete}$, and cultivated under standard growth conditions. Supernatants and cells were collected at different time points and stored at -80°C. Viral RNA was isolated and quantified by real-time RT-PCR. Chemokine induction was monitored by ELISA. HIV co-infections were performed 48 hours post GBV-C infection.

### 7.8.2. Gene Transfer into Human T Cells by Herpesvirus saimiri
*Herpesvirus saimiri* (HVS) is the classical prototype of gamma-2-herpesviruses or rhadinoviruses and persists in T lymphocytes of its natural host without any obvious disease. Whereas HVS is apathogenic in squirrel monkeys, experimental HVS infection of other primate species induces acute peripheral T cell lymphomas. Based on the pathogenic phenotype and extensive sequence variation in the N-terminus of the L-DNA of the HVS genome, virus strains were classified into the subgroups A, B, and C[84]. Subtype C strain C488 is able to transform human T cells, which harbors then multiple copies of the HVS genome in form of stable, non-integrated episomes[23]. HVS$_{C488}$ transformed T lymphocytes maintain the antigenic specificity and other functions of their parenteral T cell clone, express only a few viral proteins, and did not produce HVS virions. Therefore, *HVS* is a suitable tool for gene transfer into human T cells.

**Manufacture of GBV-C Expression Plasmids**
Overlapping GBV-C gene fragments were cloned between the CMV promoter and the poly A signal of pRSETB_P$_{CMV}$ considering the ORF of GBV-C. The BsiWI-AvrII (BA) fragment of pCR2.1_AF121950, coding for the E1-E2-p5.6-NS2-NS3$_{aa1-282}$ (nt328-4070), was inserted into the BsiWI (nt989) and AvrII (nt1040) restriction site of pRSETB_P$_{CMV}$ generating pRSETB_P$_{CMV}$_BA representing the N-terminal part of the GBV-C genome. The Eco47III-SgrAI (ES) fragment coding for the NS2$_{aa187-253}$-NS3-NS4A-NS4B-NS5A$_{aa1-61}$ (nt3037-6336), was inserted into the Eco47III (nt1025) and SgrAI (nt1049) restriction site of pRSETB_P$_{CMV}$ generating the vector pRSETB_P$_{CMV}$_ES. The Eco47III-BamHI$_{MCS}$ (EB) fragment coding for the NS2$_{aa187-253}$-NS3-NS4A-NS4B-NS5A-NS5B (nt3037-9395), was inserted into the Eco47III (nt1025) and BamHI (nt1036) restriction site of pRSETB_P$_{CMV}$ generating the expression vector pRSETB_pCMV_EB representing the C-terminal part of the GBV-C genome.

**Manufacture of HVS$_{GBV-C}$ Cosmids**
The SwaI fragments of each pRSETB_P$_{CMV}$ vector coding for the GBV-C expression cassette GBV-C$_{E1-NS2}$ (BA), GBV-C$_{NS3-NS4B}$ (ES) or GBV-C$_{NS3-NS5B}$ (EB) were cloned between the SwaI restriction sites of cosmid cos331. Hereby, the insert could be integrated in sense or anti-sense orientation generating the cosmids cos331-BA, cos331-BArev, cos331-ESrev, cos331-EB, or cos331-EBrev. Cosmid cos331 represents the N-terminal part of the HVS genome and is part of a set of five overlapping cosmids (cos331, cos261, cos291, cos336, cosDc5) that encode the entire genome of HVS$_{C488}$.

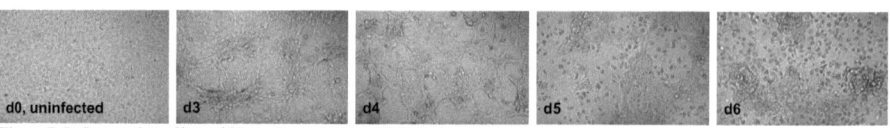
Figure 7-5: Cytopathic effect of *Herpesvirus saimiri* on OMK cells.

**Production of HVS$_{GBV-C}$ Chimeras and Transformation of Human Lymphocytes**
To produce infectious HVS$_{GBV-C}$ particles bearing the different GBV-C gene cassettes, low-passage (<30) OMK cells were co-transfected with cos331-BA, cos331-BArev, cos331-ESrev, cos-331-EB or cos331-EBrev and the other cosmids of the HVS$_{C488}$ cosmid set. The day before transfection, 6x10$^5$ OMK cells were sowed in 25cm$^2$ flasks in DMEM$_{complete}$ without antibiotics, so that they were 50-90% confluent on the next day. Per well, 0.3µg of each NotI linearized and phenol/chloroform purified cosmid were diluted in OptiMEM™ to a final volume of 292.5µl, mixed with 7.5µl of Lipofectamine™, and incubated at room temperature for 30 minutes. The cell culture medium was removed and cells were washed in OptiMEM™ prior 1.5ml fresh OptiMEM™ and 300µl of the respective DNA-Lipofectamine™ mixture were added. The transfection mix was removed six hours later. HVS$_{GBV-C}$ chimeras (HVS$_{GBV-C\_E1-NS2}$, HVS$_{GBV-C\_E1-NS2rev}$, HVS$_{GBV-C\_NS3-NS4Brev}$, HVS$_{GBV-C\_NS3-NS5B}$, HVS$_{GBV-C\_NS3-NS5Brev}$) reassembled via homologous recombination. Production of chimeric viruses is indicated by a cytopathic effect. Supernatants were collected and used to produce virus stocks by infection of fresh OMK cells. Therefore, 100% confluent 25cm$^2$ cell culture flasks were split 1:2 and cultivated for 3 days prior the medium was aspirated and cells were covered with 1ml DMEM$_{complete}$ and 500µl of HVS$_{GBV-C}$ containing supernatant. Infection was performed for 1 hour at 37°C. Cells were washed and cultivated as described before. After several days a HVS mediated cytopathic effect was visible (Figure 7-5) and virus containing supernatant was collected, filtered through a 0.22µm filter, and stored at 4°C for immediate use or was frozen at -80°C for long-term storage. HVS DNA was extracted and viral load was quantified by real-time PCR.

### 7.8.3. HIV-1 Infection Assays

**Production of HIV-1 Virus Stocks**
HIV-1 strains were cultivated on PBMC, PM1, CEMx174, and CEMx174$_{CCR5}$ cells. Therefore, 2x10$^7$ cells were infected for 4 hours at 37° in a humidified incubator with an MOI of 10 of the respective HIV-1 isolate prior cells were washed and cultivated in 20ml RPMI$_{complete}$. Ongoing replication of CXCR4-tropic HIV-1 strains was observed by syncytia formation. When a strong CPE became visible, cells were resuspended in 10ml of fresh RPMI$_{complete}$. 24 hours later the supernatant was collected, filtered through a 0.22µm filter, and aliquots were stored at -80°C. Infection of CCR5-tropic HIV strains were monitored by p24 ELISA. High titer supernatants were collected, filtered, and stored at -80°C. Virus stocks of laboratory HIV-1 strains were produced by infection of target cells with supernatants of 293T cells that were transfected with proviral DNA of the respective HIV-1 strain.

**TCID$_{50}$ and MOI**
The Tissue Culture Infectious Dose 50 (TCID$_{50}$) is defined as that dilution required to infect 50% of the cell cultures. The multiplicity of infection (MOI) is the ratio defined by the average number of virus particles deposited in a well divided by the number of target cells present in

$$\text{proportionate distance} = \frac{(\% \text{ positives above } 50\%) - 50\%}{(\% \text{ positives above } 50\%) - (\% \text{ positives below } 50\%)}$$

$$\log \text{TCID}_{50} = (\text{proportionate distance} \times \log \text{dilution factor}) + (\log \text{dilution above } 50\%)$$

Figure 7-6: Calculation of the $\text{TCID}_{50}$.

that well. $5 \times 10^4$ target cells in 100µl $\text{RPMI}_{complete}$ were sowed per well of a 96well plate. The virus stock was thawed rapidly and 10-fold virus dilutions ($10^{-3}$-$10^{-9}$) in $\text{RPMI}_{complete}$ were prepared. Per dilution, replicates of 12 were infected with 100µl/well, mixed, and incubated at 37°C. To calculate the $\text{TCID}_{50}$ of wildtype HIV, CPE development was recorded and p24 antigen concentration was measured at day 10. $\text{TCID}_{50}$ of $\text{HIV}_{PP}$ were determined by luciferase activity in the cell lysates 3 days post infection.

**Infection with Wildtype HIV-1 Strains**

$2 \times 10^6$ cells were infected for 4 hours at 37°C with an MOI of 1-8, corresponding to 25ng p24 for CCR5-tropic and 0.5ng p24 for CXCR4- and dual-tropic HIV-1 isolates in a total volume of 500µl $\text{RPMI}_{complete}$. Cells were washed, resuspended in the respective, conditioned growth medium, and cultivated for up to 2 weeks. HIV replication was monitored by p24.

**Single Round of Infection Assay using HIV-1 Pseudoparticles**

PBMC, CEMx174, CEMx174$_{CCR5}$, and TZM-bl cells were adjusted to to $5 \times 10^6$/ml, $1 \times 10^5$/ml, and $5 \times 10^5$/ml, respectively. 100µl cell suspension were sowed per well of a 96well plate and infected with 50µl of $\text{HIV}_{PP}$ (MOI of 0.1-1). Luciferase activity was measured in the cell lysates three days later.

### 7.8.4. Plaque Assays

Plaque forming units (pfu) of Adenovirus (Ad) type 5 and 12 as well as of the Yellow fever virus (YFV) strain 17D were determined in 6well plates on BHK-21$_{CAR}$ and Vero-B4 cells, respectively. Confluent cell monolayers were washed and 1ml of virus suspension was adsorbed for 1 hour at 37°C in a humidified incubator prior the inoculum was removed and cells were covered with 3ml of DMEM/10% FBS/1% agar supplemented with 350µg/ml L-glutamine and 100µg/ml gentamycin. After 4 days, the plates were overlaid with 2ml plaque medium supplemented with 0.0025% neutral red. 4 days later plaques were counted and pfu/ml were calculated.

## 7.9. Immuno Assays

### 7.9.1. Detection of anti-E2 Antibodies

GBV-C E2 directed antibodies were detected by the µ-Plate anti-HGenv ELISA (Roche Diagnostics, Penzberg) according to manufactures protocol.

### 7.9.2. Detection of Viral and Recombinant GBV-C E2 Proteins

To detect recombinant E2 protein, 16µl of the protein sample and of respective controls were diluted with 64µl incubation buffer I, incubated for 30 minutes, mixed with 20µl of a 1:20 dilution of human anti-E2 positive serum, and subjected to the µPlate anti-HGenv ELISA.

### 7.9.3. Detection of HIV-1 specific Antibodies

HIV-1 specific antibodies were detected by the AxSYM HIV Ag/Ab Combo (Abbott Diagnostics, Wiesbaden) according to manufactures protocol.

### 7.9.4. Quantification of the HIV p24 Antigen

Concentration of p24 antigen was quantified by the Murex HIV Antigen mAb ELISA (Abbott, Wiesbaden) according to manufactures protocol.

### 7.9.5. Membrane Lipid Array

Membranes with spotted lipids (Mobitec, Göttingen) were covered with PBS/1% non-fat dried milk and agitate overnight at room temperature. Blocking solution was removed and membrane was incubated for 1 hour at room temperature with 2 µg/ml anti-E2, anti-gp41, or anti-gp120 antibodies diluted in PBS/2% FBS. Then, the strip was washed twice in PBS/2% FBS/0.1% Tween-20 and incubated for 1 hour at room temperature with rabbit anti-human HRP or goat anti-mouse HRP (Dako, Hamburg) prior the membrane was analyzed via chemiluminescence.

## 7.10. Immunohistochemistry

### 7.10.1. Immunofluorescence

$5x10^5$ 293T cells were sowed on slides (Medco, Munich) and fixed in 4% PFA or in acetone/methanol for 1 hour at 4°C prior the slides were washed in PBS/2% FBS/0.1% Tween-20. To stain cell surface structures, each dot was covered for 1 hour at 4°C with 20µl of a 100µg/ml antibody dilution that was prepared in PBS/2% FBS. The slides were washed in PBS/2% FBS/0.1% Tween-20 and stained for 1 hour at 4°C with an appropriate fluorescent dye conjugated secondary antibody diluted in PBS/2% FBS. For intracellular staining, cells were fixed and permeabilized for 10-15 minutes in PBS/2% FBS/0.2% saponine. In addition, antibody dilutions contained 0.2% of saponine. Finally, the slides were washed in PBS/2% FBS/0.1% Tween-20 and mounted in DABCO/Mowiol (Sigma-Aldrich, Taufkirchen).

### 7.10.2. Flow Cytometry

Cells were washed in PBS/2% FBS and adjusted to $2x10^7$ cells/ml. For extracellular staining, 50µl of cell suspension were mixed with 50µl of antibody prepared in PBS/2% FBS, incubated for 1 hour at 4°C, and washed in PBS/2% FKS prior staining for 30 minutes at 4°C with 50µl of an appropriate fluorescent dye conjugated secondary antibody was performed. Cells were washed, resuspended in PBS, and analyzed on a FACSCalibur™ flow cytometer (BD Biosciences, Heidelberg). For intracellular staining, PFA-fixed cells were permeabilized for 10-15 minutes at 4°C with 0.2% saponine in PBS/2% FBS, washed twice, and incubated with the respective primary antibody diluted in PBS/2% FBS/0.2% saponine for 1 hour at 4°C.

### 7.10.3. Fluorescence Activated Cell Sorting

Green fluorescent Tet-Off cells were harvested, washed, and diluted in PBS/2% FBS/1mM EDTA to a final concentration of $1x10^6$ cells/ml. Cell sorting was performed at the Nikolaus-Fiebiger centre for molecular medicine of the University Erlangen-Nuremberg.

## 7.11. Polymerase Chain Reactions

### 7.11.1. Molecular Cloning of Recombinant Proteins

GBV-C sequences were amplified in a one-step RT-PCR using gene specific oligonucleotide primers and the SuperScript III One-Step RT-PCR System with Platinum Hifi Taq (Invitrogen, Groningen). Plasmid DNA was amplified by the Phusion High-Fidelity PCR Kit (New England Biolabs, Frankfurt/Main). Amplicons size (Table 7-8; coding sequence + additional nt) were analyzed by gel electrophoresis. PCR products were purified by the QIAquick Gel Extraction or PCR Purification Kit (Qiagen, Hilden) prior digestion and ligation was performed.

| protein | sequence of the respective isolate/vector | annealing temperature | elongation time | size of the amplicon |
|---|---|---|---|---|
| GBV-C E1 | AF121950: nt555-1166 | 69.0°C | 10s | 612 + 33bp |
| GBV-C E2 | AF121950: nt1167-2318 | 65.5°C | 18s | 1152 + 26bp |
| GBV-C E2(340) | AF121950: nt1164-2184 | 72.0°C | 16s | 1021 + 27bp |
| GBV-C p5.6 | AF121950: nt2319-2477 | 70.1°C | 3s | 159 + 26bp |
| GBV-C NS2 | AF121950: nt2478-3236 | 70.0°C | 12s | 759 + 41bp |
| GBV-C NS3 | AF121950: nt3237-5201 | 65.5°C | 30s | 1965 + 38bp |
| GBV-C NS4A | AF121950: nt5202-5834 | 65.5°C | 10s | 633 + 40bp |
| GBV-C NS4B | AF121950: nt5835-6155 | 68.0°C | 5s | 321 + 40bp |
| GBV-C NS5A | AF121950: nt6153-7391 | 62.8°C | 19s | 1236 + 40bp |
| GBV-C NS5B | AF121950: nt7392-9080 | 67.5°C | 26s | 1692 + 31bp |
| signal peptide Epoetin | pcDNA3-E2TM: nt994-1030 | 66.7°C | 3s | 87 + 44bp |
| c-myc/His | pCEP4-Fc: nt10351-10413rev | 65.0°C | 2s | 63 + 41bp |

Table 7-8: Amplification characteristics of selected proteins for High Fidelity PCR using the Phusion polymerase.

### 7.11.2. Colony PCR

To screen for positive *E. coli* clones, selected colonies were picked with a sterile pipette tip and inserted into the PCR master mix, PCR was conducted and amplicons were analyzed by agarose gel electrophoresis.

| reaction mix | | thermal cycle conditions | | | |
|---|---|---|---|---|---|
| water (PCR grade) | 6.45µl | temperature control: | tube | | |
| reaction buffer, 10x | 1.00µl | temperature of the lid: | 98°C/wait | | |
| dNTP, 1.25mM | 1.50µl | 1_initial Denaturation | 98°C | 10 min. | |
| 5' primer, 10µM | 0.50µl | 2_Denaturation | 98°C | 1 min | |
| 3' primer, 10µM | 0.50µl | 3_Annealing | 60 – 72°C | 30 sec. | |
| AmpliTaq, 5U/µl | 0.05µl | 4_Extension | 72°C | 1 min./kbp | 30x |
| | 10.0µl | | 4°C | hold | |

Table 7-9: Reaction mix and thermal cycle conditions for colony PCR.

### 7.11.3. Quantification of Viral DNA by Real-Time PCR

Viral DNA was extracted from 200µl sample and eluted in 100µl water using the MagNA Pure LC DNA Isolation Kit I (Roche Diagnostics, Mannheim) according to manufactures protocol. DNA was quantified by real-time PCR using a AbiPrism® 7000 or 7500.

## Quantification of Adenovirus DNA

Primer (ADP1s: nt245-269, AQ1as: nt376-354) and probe (FAM-ADO: nt313-285) are located in the hexon gene of the Ad-5 isolate X02997). Real-time PCR (Table 7-10) was conducted to quantify Adenovirus DNA.

| reaction mix | | thermal cycle conditions | | | |
|---|---|---|---|---|---|
| TaqMan® Universal PCR Master Mix (Applied Biosystems, Darmstadt) contains AmpliTaq Gold® DNA Polymerase, AmpErase®UNG, and the passive reference dye ROX in an optimized buffer. | | 5' ADP1s: | 5'-GCC GCA GTG GTC TTA CAT GCA CAT C-3' | | |
| | | 3' AQ1as: | 5'-GCC ACG GTG GGG TTT CTA AAC TT-3' | | |
| | | probe: | 5'-FAM-TGC ACC AGA CCC GGG CTC AGG TAC TCC GA-TAMRA-3' | | |
| water (PCR grade) | 5.0µl | | | | |
| master mix, 2x | 25.0µl | 1_UNG Treatment | 50°C | 2 min. | |
| 5' ADP1s, 10µM | 4.5µl | 2_initial Denaturation | 95°C | 10 min | |
| 3' AQ1as, 10µM | 4.5µl | 3_Denaturation | 95°C | 20 sec. | |
| FAM-ADO, 10µM | 1.0µl | 4_Annealing | 55°C | 20 sec. | |
| DNA extract | 10.0µl | 5_Extension | 65°C | 1 min. | 45x |

Table 7-10: Reaction mix and thermal cycle conditions to quantify Adenovirus DNA.

## Quantification of Herpesvirus saimiri DNA

Primer (5'HVS: nt45251-45275, 3'HVS: nt45357-45334) and probe (VIC-HVS: nt45324-45298) are located in the major capsid protein, ORF 25 of HVS (GenBank accession number: GI 30348501). Real-time PCR (Table 7-11) was conducted to quantify HVS DNA.

| reaction mix | | thermal cycle conditions | | | |
|---|---|---|---|---|---|
| TaqMan® Universal PCR Master Mix (Applied Biosystems, Darmstadt) contains AmpliTaq Gold® DNA Polymerase, AmpErase®UNG, and the passive reference dye ROX in an optimized buffer. | | 5' HVS: | 5'-CTC ATT ACC AGA CCC ATG TTA TGA A-3' | | |
| | | 3' HVS: | 5'-CCA TTT GCC TGT GTT GAG AGT TAA-3' | | |
| | | probe: | 5'-VIC-CTC CGA GAG AGC CTA TCT GAG ATG CCC-TAMRA -3' | | |
| water (PCR grade) | 10.0µl | | | | |
| master mix, 2x | 25.0µl | 1_UNG Treatment | 50°C | 2 min. | |
| 5' HVS, 5µM | 2.0µl | 2_initial Denaturation | 95°C | 10 min | |
| 3' HVS, 5µM | 2.0µl | 3_Denaturation | 95°C | 10 sec. | |
| VIC-HVS, 10µM | 1.0µl | 4_Annealing/ | | | |
| DNA extract | 10.0µl | Extension | 65°C | 1 min. | 45x |

Table 7-11: Reaction mix and thermal cycle conditions to quantify *Herpesvirus saimiri* DNA.

### 7.11.4. Quantification of Viral RNA by Real-Time RT-PCR

Viral RNA was extracted from 140µl sample by the QIAamp Viral RNA Mini Kit (Qiagen, Hilden), eluted in 30µl elution buffer, and was quantified by real-time RT-PCR.

| reaction mix | | thermal cycle conditions | | | |
|---|---|---|---|---|---|
| SuperScript III Platinum One-Step Quantitative RT-PCR | | 5' YFV: | 5'-AAC CCA CAC ATG CAG GAC AA-3' | | |
| water (PCR grade) | 8.5µl | 3' YFV: | 5'-GTT GCA GGT CAG CAT CCA CA-3' | | |
| reaction mix, 2x | 25.0µl | probe: | 5'-FAM-CCA TTT AGT CAT CCA TCG TAT CCG AAC GC-TAMRA-3' | | |
| 5' YFV, 10µM | 1.5µl | | | | |
| 3' YFV, 10µM | 1.5µl | 1_RT | 55°C | 30 min. | |
| FAM$_{YFV}$, 10µM | 2.0µl | 2_initial Denaturation | 95°C | 3 min | |
| ROX, 25µM | 0.5µl | 3_Denaturation | 95°C | 30 sec. | |
| RT/Taq | 1.0µl | 4_Annealing/ | | | |
| RNA extract | 10.0µl | Extension | 60°C | 60 sec. | 45x |

Table 7-12: Reaction mix and thermal cycle conditions to quantify YFV RNA (SuperScript III One-Step qRT-PCR kit).

## Quantification of YFV RNA

Primer (5'YFV: nt:10109-10128, 3'YVF: nt10337-10318) and probe (FAM-YFV: nt10237-10266) are located in the 3' UTR of $YVF_{17D}$ (GenBank accession number: X03700). PCR was performed using the SuperScript III Platinum One-Step qRT-PCR system (Table 7-12; Invitrogen, Groningen) described before[13].

## Quantification of GBV-C RNA

GBV-C was quantified using the SuperScript III Platinum One-Step qRT-PCR system (Table 7-13) or the Platinum qRT-PCR ThermoScript One-Step (Table 7-14; Invitrogen, Groningen).

| reaction mix | | thermal cycle conditions | | | |
|---|---|---|---|---|---|
| Platinum Quantitative RT-PCR ThermoScript One-Step | | | | | |
| water (PCR grade) | 2.6µl | 5' GBV-C: | 5'-GGC GAC CGG CCA AAA-3' | | |
| reaction mix, 2x | 10.0µl | 3' GBV-C: | 5'-CTT AAG ACC CAC CTA TAG TGG CTA CC-3' | | |
| 5' GBV-C, 10µM | 0.6µl | probe: | 5'-FAM-TGA CCG GGA TTT ACG ACC TAC CAA CC CT -TAMRA-3' | | |
| 3' GBV-C, 10µM | 0.6µl | 1_RT | 55°C | 30 min. | |
| $FAM_{GBV-C}$, 10µM | 0.4µl | 2_initial Denaturation | 95°C | 5 min | |
| ROX, 25µM | 0.4µl | 3_Denaturation | 95°C | 15 sec. | |
| RT/Taq | 0.4µl | 4_Annealing/ | | | |
| RNA extract | 5.0µl | Extension | 60°C | 1 min. | 40x |

Table 7-13: Reaction mix and thermal cycle conditions to quantify GBV-C RNA (ThermoScript One-Step qRT-PCR kit).

| reaction mix | | thermal cycle conditions | | | |
|---|---|---|---|---|---|
| SuperScript III Platinum One-Step Quantitative RT-PCR | | | | | |
| water (PCR grade) | 3.0µl | 5' GBV-C: | 5'-GGC GAC CGG CCA AAA-3' | | |
| reaction mix, 2x | 10.0µl | 3' GBV-C: | 5'-CTT AAG ACC CAC CTA TAG TGG CTA CC-3' | | |
| 5' GBV-C, 10µM | 0.4µl | probe: | 5'-FAM-TGA CCG GGA TTT ACG ACC TAC CAA CC CT-TAMRA-3' | | |
| 3' GBV-C, 10µM | 0.4µl | 1_RT | 55°C | 15 min. | |
| $FAM_{GBV-C}$, 10µM | 0.4µl | 2_initial Denaturation | 95°C | 2 min | |
| ROX, 25µM | 0.4µl | 3_Denaturation | 95°C | 15 sec. | |
| RT/Taq | 0.4µl | 4_Annealing/ | | | |
| RNA extract | 5.0µl | Extension | 60°C | 33 sec. | 40x |

Table 7-14: Reaction mix and thermal cycle conditions to quantify GBV-C RNA (SuperScript III One-Step qRT-PCR kit).

# 8. Material

## 8.1. Media, Buffers, and Solutions

### 8.1.1. Media, Buffers, and Solutions for Prokaryotic Cell Culture

**Inoue Transformation Buffer**
10.88g $MnCl_2$-$4H_2O$, 2.20g $CaCl_2$-$2H_2O$, 18.65g KCl, and 20ml 0.5M PIPES (pH 6.7) were dissolved in 1l $H_2O_{dd}$. 0.5M PIPES were prepared by dissolving 15.1g PIPES in 80ml $H_2O_{dd}$ and adjusting of the pH to 6.7 with 5M KOH prior $H_2O_{dd}$ was added to a final volume of 100ml. The transformation buffer was filtered through a 0.45µM filter and sterile aliquots were stores at -20°C. Final concentration: 55mM $MnCl_2$, 15mM $CaCl_2$, 250mM KCl, 10mM PIPES.

**Luria-Bertani Medium**
10g peptone, 5g yeast extract, and 5g NaCl were solved in 950ml $H_2O_{Milli-Q}$, adjusted to pH 7.2 in a total volume of 1l, and sterilized by autoclaving. To prepare nutrient, selective agar plates, 1l LB medium was mixed with 16g agar, autoclaved and chilled to 50°C prior the respective antibiotic (Table 8-1) was added and 10cm dishes were filled with 20ml LB agar.

| antibiotic | ampicillin | kanamycin | tetracycline | neomycin |
|---|---|---|---|---|
| stock solution | 50mg/ml | 15mg/ml | 1mg/ml | 100mg/ml |
| final concentration | 100µg/ml | 30µg/ml | 10µg/ml | 30µg/ml |

Table 8-1: Antibiotics for prokaryotic selection.

**SOB Medium**
20g tryptone, 5g yeast extract, and 0.5g NaCl were dissolved in 950ml $H_2O_{Milli-Q}$. 10ml of a 250mM KCl solution were added and pH was adjusted to 7.0 with 5N NaOH prior the volume was adjusted to 1l. The solution was sterilized by autoclaving. Just before use, 5ml of sterile 1M $MgCl_2$ and 5ml of sterile 1M $MgSO_4$ were added.

**SOC Medium**
20g tryptone, 5g yeast extract, and 0.5g NaCl were dissolved in 950ml $H_2O_{Milli-Q}$. 10ml of a 250mM KCl solution were added and pH was adjusted to 7.0 with 5N NaOH prior the volume was adjusted to 1l. The solution was sterilized by autoclaving. Just before use, 10ml of sterile 1M $MgCl_2$, 10ml of sterile 1M $MgSO_4$, and 20ml 1M glucose (steril) were added.

**X-gal solution, 2% (w/v)**
100mg X-gal were solved in 5ml DMSO and stored light protected at -20°C.

### 8.1.2. Media, Buffers, and Solutions for Eukaryotic Cell Culture

**BES Transfection Buffer, 2x**
11.8g BES, 16.4g NaCl, and 0.21g $Na_2HPO_4$ were dissolved in 1l $H_2O_{Milli-Q}$, adjusted to pH 6.95 with 5N NaOH, and filtered through a 0.22µm filter. Aliquots were stored at -20°C. Final concentration: 50mM BES, 280mM NaCl, 1.5mM $Na_2HPO_4$.

**Calcium Chloride, 2.5M**
11g of $CaCl_2$-$6H_2O$ were dissolved in 20ml $H_2O_{dd}$ and sterilized by passing through a 0.22µm filter. Aliquots were frozen at -20°C.

## Dulbecco's Modified Eagle Medium (DMEM)
13.38g DMEM and 3.7g $NaHCO_3$ were solved in 950ml $H_2O_{Ampuwa}$, adjusted to pH 7.05 in a final volume of 1l, and sterile filtered through a 0.22µm filter. $DMEM_{complete}$ was made of 90% DMEM and 10% FBS, supplemented with 350µg/ml L-Glutamin, and 100µg/ml Gentamycin.

## Doxycycline, 10mg/ml
1g doxycycline were dissolved 100ml $H_2O_{Milli-Q}$ and sterilized by passing through a 0.22µm filter. Aliquots were frozen at -20°C and could be frozen/thawed up to five times.

## Geneticin, 50mg/ml
500mg geneticin sulfate (G418, >650U/mg) were dissolved in PBS to a final volume of 10ml and sterilized by passing through a 0.22µm filter. Aliquots were frozen at -20°C.

## HEPES Transfection Buffer, 2x
11.9g HEPES, 16.4g NaCl, and 0.21g $Na_2HPO_4$ were dissolved in 1l $H_2O_{Milli-Q}$, adjusted to pH 7.05 with 5N NaOH, and filtered through a 0.22µm filter. Aliquots were stored at -20°C. Final concentration: 50mM HEPES, 280mM NaCl, 1.5mM $Na_2HPO_4$.

## Hygromycin B, 100mg/ml
1g hygromycin B (>900U/mg) were dissolved in PBS to a final volume of 10ml and sterilized by passing through a 0.22µm filter. Stock solution was stored at 4°C.

## Methotrexate, 10mg/ml
100mg methotrexate hydrate were dissolved in a final volume of 10ml 50mM sodium carbonate buffer (pH 9.0) and sterilized by passing through a 0.22µm filter. Aliquots were stored at -20°C.

## Minimum Essential Medium (MEM)
9.6g MEM and 2.2g $NaHCO_3$ were solved in 950ml $H_2O_{Ampuwa}$, adjusted to pH 7.05 in a final volume of 1l, and sterile filtered through a 0.22µm filter.

## Phosphate Buffered Saline (PBS)
PBS0 was prepared by solving 16g NaCl, 2.3g $Na_2HPO_4$-$2H_2O$, 0.4g KCl, and 0.4g $KH_2PO_4$ in 950ml $H_2O_{Milli-Q}$, adjusted to pH 7.3 prior solution was steril filtered through a 0.22µm filter. For PBS, 4.6ml 2M $CaCl_2$ and 4.9ml $MgCl_2$ were added. Final concentration: 136.89mM NaCl, 8.10mM $Na_2HPO_4$, 2.68mM KCl, 1.46mM $KH_2PO_4$, 0.91mM $CaCl_2$, 0.91mM $MgCl_2$.

## Puromycin, 100mg/ml
1g puromycin dihydrochlorid were dissolved in PBS to a final volume of 10ml and sterilized by passing through a 0.22µm filter. Aliquots were stored at 4°C.

## Roswell Park Memorial Institute Medium (RPMI)
10.43g RPMI and 2.0g $NaHCO_3$ were solved in 950ml $H_2O_{Ampuwa}$, adjusted to pH 7.05 in a final volume of 1l, and sterilized by passing through a 0.22µm filter. $RPMI_{comple}$ was made of 40% RPMI, 50% Panserin, 10% FBS, supplemented with 350µg/ml L-glutamin and 100µg/ml gentamycin.

## Trypsin-EDTA
8g $NaCl_2$, 0.4g KCl, 0.1g $Na_2HPO_4$, 1.0g glucose, and 3.0g Tris were solved in 900ml $H_2O_{Ampuwa}$ and adjusted to pH 7.5 prior 0.1g EDTA, 1.2g trypsin, and 5ml 0.1% phenol red were added; pH was adjusted again and the volume was filled up to 1l.

## 8.1.3. Media, Buffers, and Solutions for Protein Analysis

### ATP, 0.2M
12.1g adenosine-5'-triphosphate disodium salt were dissolved in 50ml $H_2O_{Milli-Q}$ and pH was adjusted to 7.0 with 2M Tris-HCl (pH 8.8). $H_2O_{Milli-Q}$ was added to finial volume of 100ml. Aliquots were stored at -20°C.

### Cell Lysis Buffer, 2x
62.5ml 0.1M Tris-HCl (pH 7.8), 0.5ml 1M DTT, 2.5ml TritonX-100, 25ml Glycerol, and 173mg DCTA were dissolved in $H_2O_{Milli-Q}$ to finial volume of 125ml. Aliquots were stored at -20°C.

### Coomassie Blue R-250 Staining Solution
250mg Coomassie Brilliant Blue R-250 were dissolved in 10ml glacial acetic acid and diluted with 90ml of methanol:$H_2O_{Milli-Q}$ (1:2).

### Coomassie Blue G-250 Staining Solution
250mg Coomassie Brilliant Blue G-250 were dissolved in 100ml acetic acid and adjusted with $H_2O_{Milli-Q}$ to a final volume of 1l.

### Coomassie Blue Stripping Solution
50ml glacial acetic acid, 100ml methanol, and 850ml $H_2O_{Milli-Q}$ were mixed.

### Dithiothreitol, 1M
3.09g dithiothreitol were dissolved in 20ml 10mM sodium acetate (pH 5.2) and sterilized by filtration. Aliquots were stored at -20°C.

### DNA Sample Buffer, 5x
4g sucrose, 2.5mg bromophenol blue, and 2.5mg xylene cyanol were solved in 10ml PBS.

### ECL solution A
250mg luminol and 100ml 1M Tris-HCl (pH 8.6) were diluted in 1l $H_2O_{Milli-Q}$. Aliquots were stored at 4°C.

### ECL solution B
1.1mg p-coumaric acid were solved in 1ml DMSO and stored at room temperature.

### FACS Buffer
81.2g NaCl, 2.6g $KH_2PO_4$, 23.5g $Na_2HPO_4$, 2.8g KCl, 3.6g $Na_2EDTA$, and 4.3g LiCl were solved in 10l $H_2O_{Milli-Q}$ and filtered. Final concentration: 138.94mM NaCl, 1.91mM $KH_2PO_4$, 16.67mM $Na_2HPO_4$, 3.71mM KCl, 0.97mM $Na_2EDTA$, 10.14mM LiCl.

### Luciferin, 25mM
25mg D-luciferin were dissolved in 3.5ml luciferase assay buffer. Aliquots were stored at -20°C.

### Luciferase Assay Buffer
180µl 1M $MgSO_4$, 1.2ml 1M potassium phosphate buffer (pH 7.0), 0.6ml 0.2M ATP, and 120µl 25mM Luciferin were diluted in 9.9ml $H_2O_{Milli-Q}$. Final concentration: 15mM $MgSO_4$, 100mM potassium phosphate, 10mM ATP, 250µM luciferin.

### Potassium Phosphate Buffer, 1M, pH 5.8-8.0
87.1g $K_2HPO_4$ as well as 126.3g $KH_2PO_4$ were dissolved in $H_2O_{Milli-Q}$ to a final volume of 500ml. Both 1M stock solutions were mixed until the desired pH was reached (Table 8-2).

| pH: | 5.8 | 6.0 | 6.2 | 6.4 | 6.6 | 6.8 | 7.0 | 7.2 | 7.4 | 7.6 | 7.8 | 8.0 |
|---|---|---|---|---|---|---|---|---|---|---|---|---|
| 1M $K_2HPO_4$ (ml) | 8.5 | 13.2 | 19.2 | 27.8 | 38.1 | 49.7 | 61.5 | 71.7 | 80.2 | 86.6 | 90.8 | 94.0 |
| 1M $KH_2PO_4$ (ml) | 91.5 | 86.8 | 80.8 | 72.2 | 61.9 | 50.3 | 38.5 | 28.3 | 19.8 | 13.4 | 9.2 | 6.0 |

Table 8-2: Preparation of potassium phosphate buffer at 25°C.

**SDS-Page: Acetic Acid Gel Buffer, 0.2M, pH 3.7-5.6**
11.49ml glacial acetic acid were diluted with Milli-Q $H_2O$ to a final volume of 500ml, pH was adjusted with 1M NaOH, and $H_2O_{Milli-Q}$ has been added to 1l.

**SDS-Page: Glycine Gel Buffer, 0.2M, pH 8.6-10.6**
15.01g glycine were dissolved in 500ml $H_2O_{Milli-Q}$, pH was adjusted with 1M NaOH, and $H_2O_{Milli-Q}$ has been added to 1l.

**SDS-Page: Phosphate Gel Buffer, 0.2M, pH 5.8-8.0**
55.20g $NaH_2PO_4$-$H_2O$ were dissolved in 500ml $H_2O_{Milli-Q}$, pH was adjusted with 1M NaOH, and $H_2O_{Milli-Q}$ has been added to 1l.

**SDS-Page: Tris-HCl Gel Buffer, 0.2M, pH 7.1-8.9**
24.23g Tris base were dissolved in 500ml $H_2O_{Milli-Q}$, pH was adjusted with 1N HCl, and $H_2O_{Milli-Q}$ has been added to 1l.

**SDS-Page: Tris-HCl Gel Buffer, 0.5M, pH 6.8**
6.05g Tris base was dissolved in 40ml $H_2O_{Milli-Q}$ and adjusted to pH 6.8 with 1N HCl. $H_2O_{Milli-Q}$ has been added to 100ml prior the solution have been filtered through a 0.22µm filter.

**SDS-Page: Tris-HCl Gel Buffer, 1.5M, pH 8.8**
91g Tris base was dissolved in 300ml $H_2O_{Milli-Q}$ and adjusted to pH 8.8 with 1N HCl. $H_2O_{Milli-Q}$ has been added to 500ml volume prior the solution have been filtered through a 0.22µm filter.

**SDS-Page: Sodiumphosphate/Glycerol Sample Buffer, non-reducing 5x**
2g SDS, 10ml glycerol, 1mg bromphenol blue, and 3ml 1M $Na_2HPO_4$ were mixed. $H_2O_{Milli-Q}$ has been added to 20ml. Aliquots were stored at -20°C.

**SDS-Page: Sodiumphosphate/Glycerol Sample Buffer, reducing 5x**
2g SDS, 10ml glycerol, 5ml beta-mercaptoethanol, 1mg bromphenol blue, and 3ml 1M $Na_2HPO_4$ were mixed. $H_2O_{Milli-Q}$ has been added to 20ml. Aliquots were stored at -20°C.

**SDS-Page: Tris/Glycine Electrophoresis Buffer, 10x**
15.1g Tris base, 94.0g glycine, and 5.0g SDS were dissolved in 500ml $H_2O_{Milli-Q}$. Final concentration: 250mM Tris, 2.5M glycine, 1% SDS.

**SDS-Page: Tris/Glycine Transfer buffer, 10x**
30.3g Tris base and 144.1g glycine were dissolved in 1l $H_2O_{Milli-Q}$. A ready to use solution was prepared by dilution of 100ml 10x stock solution in 150ml methanol, and $H_2O_{Milli-Q}$ to 1l. Final concentration: 25mM Tris, 192mM glycine, 15% methanol.

**Sodium Acetate, 3M**
40.83g Sodium acetate-$3H_2O$ were dissolved in 80ml $H_2O_{Milli-Q}$. pH was adjusted to 5.2 with glacial acetic acid or to 7.0 with diluted acetic acid, adjusted to a final volume of 100ml, and sterilized by passing through a 0.22µm filter.

| pH: | 5.8 | 6.0 | 6.2 | 6.4 | 6.6 | 6.8 | 7.0 | 7.2 | 7.4 | 7.6 | 7.8 | 8.0 |
|---|---|---|---|---|---|---|---|---|---|---|---|---|
| 1M Na$_2$HPO$_4$ (ml) | 7.9 | 12.0 | 17.8 | 25.5 | 35.2 | 46.3 | 57.7 | 68.4 | 77.4 | 84.5 | 89.6 | 93.2 |
| 1M NaH$_2$PO$_4$ (ml) | 92.1 | 88.0 | 82.2 | 74.5 | 64.8 | 53.7 | 42.3 | 31.6 | 22.6 | 15.5 | 10.4 | 6.8 |

Table 8-3: Preparation of sodium phosphate buffer at 25°C.

**Sodium Phosphate Buffer, 1M, pH 5.8-8.0**
71.1g Na$_2$HPO$_4$ as well as 60.0g NaH$_2$PO$_4$ were dissolved in H$_2$O$_{Milli-Q}$ to a final volume of 500ml. Both 1M stock solutions were mixed until the desired pH was reached (Table 8-3).

**TAE Buffer, 50x**
To prepare a 50x stock solution 242g Tris base were dissolved in 800ml H$_2$O$_{Milli-Q}$, mixed with 57.1ml glacial acetic acid, 100ml 0.5M EDTA, and adjusted to pH 8. H$_2$O$_{Milli-Q}$ was added to a final volume of 1l.

**TE$_{1:100}$ Buffer**
1.21g Tris base and 2.92mg EDTA were dissolved in 1l H$_2$O$_{Milli-Q}$. pH was adjusted to 7.0 or 8.0. Final concentration: 10mM Tris-HCl, 0.01mM EDTA.

**TM Buffer, 5x**
30.29g Tris base and 7.32g MgSO$_4$·7H$_2$O were dissolved in 1l H$_2$O$_{Milli-Q}$ and pH was adjusted to 7.8. Final concentration: 250mM Tris-HCl, 50mM MgSO$_4$.

**Tris/Glycerol Sample Buffer, 5x**
25ml 0.5M Tris-HCl (pH 6.8), 20ml glycerol and 1mg bromphenol blue were solved in H$_2$O$_{Milli-Q}$ to a final volume of 100ml. Aliquots were stored at -20°C.

## 8.2. Cells

### 8.2.1. Escherichia coli

**DH5alpha** F- φ80*lacZ*ΔM15 Δ(*lacZYA-argF*)U169 *deo*R *rec*A1 *end*A1 *hsd*R17 (r$_k^-$, m$_k^+$) *pho*A *sup*E44 *thi-1 gyr*A96 *rel*A1 λ- (Invitrogen, Groningen).

**HB101** F- *thi-1 hsd*S20 (r$_B^-$, m$_B^-$) *sup*E44 *rec*A13 *ara-14 leu*B6 *pro*A2 *lac*Y1 *gal*K2 *rps*L20 (Str$^R$) *xyl-5 mtl-1* (Promega, Mannheim).

**LE392** *hsd*R514(r$_k^-$, m$_k^+$), *gln*V(*sup*E44), *try*T (*sup*F58), *lac*Y1 or Δ(*lac*IZY)6, *gal*K2, *gal*T22, *met*B1, *trp*R55 (Promega, Mannheim).

**Stbl2** F- *mcr*A Δ(*mcr*BC-*hsd*RMS-*mrr*) *rec*A1 *end*A1 *lon gyr*A96 *thi sup*E44 *rel*A1 Δ(*lac-proAB*) λ- (Invitrogen, Groningen).

**Stbl3** F- *mcr*B *hsd*S20 (r$_B^-$, m$_B^-$) *sup*E44 *rec*A13 *ara-14 pro*A2 *lac*Y1 *gal*K2 *rps*L20(Str$^R$) *xyl-5 mtl-1* λ- (Invitrogen, Groningen).

**TOP10** F- φ80*lacZ*ΔM15 *mcr*A Δ*lac*X74 *rec*A1 *ara*D139 Δ(*ara, leu*) 7697 *gal*U *gal*K *rps*L (Str$^R$) *end*A1 Δ(*mrr-hsd*RMS-*mcr*BC) *nup*G (Invitrogen, Groningen).

**XL1-Blue** *lac* [F' *pro*AB *lac*I$^q$ZΔM15 Tn*10* (Tet$^R$)] *rec*A1 *end*A1 *gyr*A96 *thi-1 hsd*R17 *sup*E44 *rel*A1 (Agilent, Waldbronn).

## 8.2.2. Mammalian Cell Lines

| | |
|---|---|
| 293T | clonal derivate of the human fibroblastoid cell line 293, originally derived from a adenovirus type 5 transformed human primary embryonal kidney that carries a plasmid containing the temperature sensitive mutant of SV-40 large T-antigen[232]. Obtained from Dr. Hauke Walter, University Hospital Erlangen, Germany. |
| BHK-21$_{CAR}$ | fibroblast cell line expressing the coxsackie B virus-Ad receptor (CAR), parenteral clone was established from the kidney of a 1-day-old newborn Syrian golden hamster. Obtained from Stefanie Weber and Dr. Walter Dörfler, University Hospital Erlangen, Germany. |
| Bjab | human B lymphoblastoid cell line, established from a patient with Burkitt's lymphoma that does not contain EBV DNA[114]. Obtained from Dr. Klaus Korn, University Hospital Erlangen, Germany. |
| CEMx174 | hybrid of the human T lymphoblastoid cell line CEM and the human B lymphoblastoid cell line 721.174[240]. Obtained from Prof. Stefan Pöhlmann, University of Hanover, Germany. |
| CEMx174$_{CCR5}$ | clonal derivate of the CEMx174 cell line expressing the human CC receptor 5[175]. Obtained from Prof. Stefan Pöhlmann, University of Hanover, Germany. |
| CHO dhfr⁻ | dihydrofolate reductase-deficient subclone from the parental CHO cell line initiated from a biopsy of an ovary of an adult Chinese hamster[227,296]. Obtained from the DSMZ, Braunschweig, Germany. |
| HeLa | human epithelial-like cell line established from the cervical epithelial carcinoma of a 31-year-old female[172]. Obtained from Dr. Richard Axel through the AIDS Research and Reference Reagent Program, Division of AIDS, NIAID, NIH. |
| HeLa CD4⁺ | clone 1022, generated by infection of the parenteral HeLa cell line with a retroviral vector expressing CD4 and Neo$^R$[172]. Obtained from Dr. Bruce Chesebro through the AIDS Research and Reference Reagent Program, Division of AIDS, NIAID, NIH. |
| Jurkat$_{clone\ E6-1}$ | human T lymphoblastoid cell line, established from the peripheral blood of a 14-year-old boy with acute lymphoblastic leukemia[253,306]. Obtained from Dr. Arthur Weiss through the AIDS Research and Reference Reagent Program, Division of AIDS, NIAID, NIH. |
| Molt-4$_{clone\ 8}$ | human T cell line originally derived from the peripheral blood of a 19-year-old male with acute lymphoblastic leukemia in relapse. Clone 8 was generated by subcloning in soft agarose by Kikukawa *et al.*[63,143]. Obtained from Prof. Ronald Desrosiers through the AIDS Research and Reference Reagent Program, Division of AIDS, NIAID, NIH. |
| OMK | epithelial cell line, established from the kidney of a normal adult female Owl monkey[192]. Obtained from Dr. Bernhard Fleckenstein, University Hospital Erlangen, Germany. |

| | |
|---|---|
| P3HR-1 | human B lymphoblastoid cell line, established from an EBV-positive Burkitt's lymphoma of a 7-year-old black African boy[147]. Obtained from Dr. Klaus Korn, University Hospital Erlangen, Germany. |
| PM1 | clonal derivative of the human cutaneous T cell lymphoma cell line HUT 78 that was originally derived from the peripheral blood of a patient with Sezary syndrome[170]. Obtained from Dr. Marvin Reitz through the AIDS Research and Reference Reagent Program, Division of AIDS, NIAID, NIH. |
| Raji | human B lymphoblastoid cell line, established from an EBV-positive Burkitt's lymphoma of an 11-year-old black African boy[311]. Obtained from Dr. Klaus Korn, University Hospital Erlangen, Germany. |
| TZM-bl | previously designated as JC53-bl$_{clone\ 13}$, clonal derivate of the HeLa cell line JC.53, which expresses large amounts of CD4 and CCR5. The TZM-bl cell line was generated by introducing separate integrated copies of the luciferase and ß-galactosidase genes under control of the HIV-1 promoter[225]. Obtained from Dr. John C. Kappes, Dr. Xiaoyun Wu, and Tranzyme Inc. through the NIH AIDS Research and Reference Reagent Program, Division of AIDS, NIAID, NIH. |
| Vero-B4 | adherent-elongated, fibroblast-like cell line, established from the kidney of a normal adult African green monkey[319]. Obtained from Dr. Klaus Korn, University Hospital Erlangen, Germany. |

## 8.3. Antibodies and Normal Sera

| Antibody | Clone | Catalog number | Distributor |
|---|---|---|---|
| Mouse α-GBV-C E2 | 125 | C65520M | Biodesign, Saco, USA |
| Mouse α-GBV-C E2 | M03 | | A. Engel, Roche Diagnostics, Penzberg |
| Mouse α-GBV-C E2 | M05 | | A. Engel, Roche Diagnostics, Penzberg |
| Mouse α-GBV-C E2 | M06 | | A. Engel, Roche Diagnostics, Penzberg |
| Mouse α-GBV-C E2 | M11 | | A. Engel, Roche Diagnostics, Penzberg |
| Mouse α-GBV-C E2 | M13 | | A. Engel, Roche Diagnostics, Penzberg |
| Mouse α-GBV-C E2 | M17 | | A. Engel, Roche Diagnostics, Penzberg |
| Mouse α-GBV-C E2 | M19 | | A. Engel, Roche Diagnostics, Penzberg |
| Mouse α-GBV-C E2 | M30 | | A. Engel, Roche Diagnostics, Penzberg |
| Rabbit α-GBV-C E2 | 64236 | | J. Stapleton, Univ. of Iowa, Iowa, USA |
| Rabbit α-GBV-C E2 | B2963 | | J. Stapleton, Univ. of Iowa, Iowa, USA |
| Goat α-GBV-C NS3 | | sc-17535 | Santa Cruz Biotech., Heidelberg |
| Goat α-GBV-C NS3 | | sc-17536 | Santa Cruz Biotech., Heidelberg |
| Rabbit α-GBV-C NS5A | 64620 | | J. Stapleton, Univ. of Iowa, Iowa, USA |
| Rabbit α-GBV-C NS5A | 64631 | | J. Stapleton, Univ. of Iowa, Iowa, USA |
| Rabbit α-GBV-C NS5A | | GTC70318 | Dunn Labortechnik, Asbach |
| Rabbit α-GBV-C NS5B | 64244 | | J. Stapleton, Univ. of Iowa, Iowa, USA |
| Rabbit α-GBV-C NS5B | 64632 | | J. Stapleton, Univ. of Iowa, Iowa, USA |
| human α-HIV gp120 | 17b | 4091 | NIH AIDS Program, USA |
| human α-HIV gp120 | B4e8 | 7626 | NIH AIDS Program, USA |
| Mouse α-HIV gp120/160 | ID6 | 2343 | NIH AIDS Program, USA |
| Mouse α-hCCL3 | 93321 | MAB270 | R&D Systems, Abingdon, USA |
| Mouse α-hCCL4 | 24006 | MAB271 | R&D Systems, Abingdon, USA |

| Antibody | Clone | Catalog number | Distributor |
|---|---|---|---|
| Mouse α-hCCL5 | 21445 | MAB278 | R&D Systems, Abingdon, USA |
| Mouse α-hCXCL12 | 79014 | MAB310 | R&D Systems, Abingdon, USA |
| Mouse α-hCD4 | B4 | 7629 | NIH AIDS Program, USA |
| Mouse α-hCD4 | SIM.4 | 724 | NIH AIDS Program, USA |
| Mouse α-hCD4 FITC | RPA-T4 | 555346 | Becton Dickinson, Heidelberg |
| Mouse α-hCD4 PE | SK1 | 347327 | Becton Dickinson, Heidelberg |
| Mouse α-hCD4 PE | SK3 | 345769 | Becton Dickinson, Heidelberg |
| Mouse α-hCD4 PE | RPA-T4 | 555347 | Becton Dickinson, Heidelberg |
| Mouse α-hCD8 FITC | HIT8a | 555634 | Becton Dickinson, Heidelberg |
| Mouse α-hCD8 PE | SK1 | 345773 | Becton Dickinson, Heidelberg |
| Mouse α-hCD8 Beads | | 130-045-201 | Miltenyi Biotech, Bergisch Gladbach |
| Mouse α-hCD19 Beads | | 130-050-301 | Miltenyi Biotech, Bergisch Gladbach |
| Mouse α-hCD19 PE | 4G7 | 349209 | Becton Dickinson, Heidelberg |
| Mouse α-hCD32 | 3D3 | 551900 | Becton Dickinson, Heidelberg |
| Mouse α-hCD81 | JS-81 | 555675 | Becton Dickinson, Heidelberg |
| Mouse α-hCD81 PE | JS-81 | 555676 | Becton Dickinson, Heidelberg |
| Mouse α-hCD184 | 12G5 | 3439 | NIH AIDS Program, USA |
| Mouse α-hCD184 PE | 12G5 | 555974 | Becton Dickinson, Heidelberg |
| Mouse α-hCD195 | 2D7 | 3933 | NIH AIDS Program, USA |
| Mouse α-hCD195 PE | 2D7 | 555993 | Becton Dickinson, Heidelberg |
| Mouse α-(HIS)$_6$ | 13/45/31 | DIA900 | Dianova, Hamburg |
| Goat α-mouse IgG FITC | | 115-097-103 | Jackson IR, West Grove, USA |
| Goat α-mouse IgG HRP | | P 0447 | Dako, Hamburg |
| Goat α-mouse IgG$_1$ PE | | 1070-09S | SouthernBiotech, Birmingham, UK |
| Goat α-mouse IgG$_{2b}$ PE | | 1090-09S | SouthernBiotech, Birmingham, UK |
| Goat α-rabbit IgG FITC | | 111-095-144 | Jackson IR, West Grove, USA |
| Goat α-rabbit IgG HRP | | P 0448 | Dako, Hamburg |
| Rabbit α-goat IgG PE | | sc-3755 | Santa Cruz Biotech., Heidelberg |
| Rabbit α-goat IgG HRP | | sc-2768 | Santa Cruz Biotech., Heidelberg |
| Rabbit α-human IgG FITC | | F 0202 | Dako, Hamburg |
| Rabbit α-human IgG HRP | | P 0214 | Dako, Hamburg |
| Mouse IgG$_1$ isotype control | | P01102M | Biodesign, Saco, USA |
| Mouse IgG$_1$ isotype control | 11711 | MAB002 | R&D Systems, Abingdon, USA |
| Mouse IgG$_1$ isotype control | MOPC21 | 555746 | Becton Dickinson, Heidelberg |
| Mouse IgG$_1$ isotype control PE | MOPC21 | 554680 | Becton Dickinson, Heidelberg |
| Mouse IgG$_{2a}$ isotype control | 20102 | MAP003 | R&D Systems, Abingdon, USA |
| Mouse IgG$_{2a}$ isotype control | G155-178 | 555571 | Becton Dickinson, Heidelberg |
| Mouse IgG$_{2a}$ isotype control PE | G155-178 | 559319 | Becton Dickinson, Heidelberg |
| Mouse IgG$_{2b}$ isotype control | 20116 | MAP004 | R&D Systems, Abingdon, USA |

| Serum/Immune globuline | Catalog number | Distributor |
|---|---|---|
| normal goat serum | 005-000-121 | Dianova, Hamburg |
| normal mouse serum | 015-000-001 | Dianova, Hamburg |
| normal human serum | 009-000-121 | Dianova, Hamburg |
| human IgG | 009-000-002 | Dianova, Hamburg |

## 8.4. Plasmids

### 8.4.1. GBV-C Expression Plasmids

The GBV-C clone AF121950 was constructed by Xiang *et al.* cloning a full-length cDNA of a person with chronic GBV-C viremia into the pCR2.1 and pGEM-5ZF(-) vector[316]. Transcription by the T7 and SP6 polymerase produces full length, infectious, plus-strand as well as non-infectious, negative-strand GBV-C RNA, respectively.

**pCR2.1_Iowa[96-188]**
Constructed by amplification of nt96-188 of the GBV-C isolate AF121950 and cloning into the pCR2.1 TOPO-TA vector. T7 RNA polymerase transcribes plus-strand RNA, which is used to generate a GBV-C specific RNA standard that enables the quantification of GBV-C virus particles by real time RT-PCR.

**pCR2.1_Iowa[96-188reverse]**
Constructed by amplification of nt96-188 of the GBV-C isolate AF121950 and reverse cloning into the pCR2.1 TOPO-TA vector. T7 RNA polymerase transcribes minus-strand RNA, which is used to generate a GBV-C specific RNA standard that enables the quantification of GBV-C replication intermediates by real time RT-PCR.

**pE1-NS2$_{2626}$**
Mutant of the infectious clone pCR2.1_AF121950. Constructed by the deletion of the Eco47III/StuI fragment (nt2627-8923) and religation of the 9.8kb fragment. T7 transcribed plus-stranded RNA encodes for the viral proteins E1-E2-p5.6-NS2$_{1-50}$.

**pE1-NS4A$_{5436}$**
Mutant of the infectious clone pCR2.1_AF121950. Constructed by deletion of the StuI fragment (nt5437-8923) and religation of the 7.0kb fragment. RNA transcribed by the T7 polymerase codes for the viral proteins E1-E2-p5.6-NS2-NS3-NS4A$_{1-79}$.

**pFS**
Mutant of the infectious clone pCR2.1_AF121950. Constructed by deletion of the SnaBI fragment (nt843-4033) and religation of the 10.1kb fragment. Due to a -2nt frame shift, T7 transcribed RNA encodes only for the first 96aa of the GBV-C E1 protein.

**pCEP4_E2(340)-Fc**
Eukaryotic expression vectors encoding a soluble GBV-C E2 Fc fusion protein. Constructed by amplification of nt1164-2184 of the GBV-C isolate AF121950 or respective cDNA and ligated into the BamHI/NotI fragment of pCEP4-Fc[25,130].

**pRSETB_P$_{CMV}$_BA**
The BsiWI-AvrII (BA) fragment of pCR2.1_AF121950, coding for E1-NS3$_{aa1-282}$ (nt328-4070), was fused with the BsiWI and AvrII fragment of pRSETB_P$_{CMV}$ to generate pRSETB_P$_{CMV}$_BA. The plasmid was obtained from Dr. Jack T. Stapleton, University of Iowa, Iowa, USA.

**pRSETB_P$_{CMV}$_ES**
The Eco47III-SgrAI (ES) fragment of pCR2.1_AF121950, coding for NS2$_{aa187-253}$-NS5A$_{aa1-61}$ (nt3037-6336), was fused with the Eco47III and SgrAI fragment of pRSETB_P$_{CMV}$ to generate pRSETB_P$_{CMV}$_ES. The plasmid was obtained from Dr. Jack T. Stapleton, University of Iowa, Iowa, USA.

**pRSETB_P$_{CMV}$_EB**
The Eco47III-BamHI$_{MCS}$ (EB) fragment of pCR2.1_AF121950, coding for the NS2$_{aa187-253}$-NS5B (nt3037-9395), was fused with the Eco47III and BamHI fragment of pRSETB_P$_{CMV}$ to generate pRSETB_P$_{CMV}$_EB representing the C-terminal part of the GBV-C genome. The plasmid was obtained from Dr. Jack T. Stapleton, University of Iowa, Iowa, USA.

**pcDNA3dhfr_E2-TM**
Eukaryotic expression vector encoding the E2 protein of the GBV-C clone HGU44402. Nucleotides 1149 to 2314 of the HGV complementary DNA (GenBank accession number U44402) were subcloned into pcDNA3dhfr downstream from the signal sequence of erythropoietin and the sequence encoding for the FLAG octapaptide[278]. The plasmid was obtained from Dr. Alfred Engel, Roche Diagnostics, Penzberg, Germany.

## 8.4.2. HIV Experssion Plasmids

**pJRCSF**
Proviral full-length, replication and infection competent molecular clone of HIV-1$_{JR-CSF}$, a primary isolate from cerebral spinal fluid obtained from an AIDS patient. The plasmid was obtained from Drs. Irvin SY Chen and Yoshio Koyanagi through the NIH AIDS Research and Reference Reagent Program, Division of AIDS, NIAID, NIH.

**pYU-2**
Proviral full-length, replication and infection competent DNA of the nonpermuted HIV clone YU2. The expression vector was constructed by ligation of the 5' SalI-EcoRI and the 3' EcoRI-SphI fragment and cloning into the SphI-SalI site of pTZ19R. The plasmid was obtained from Drs. Beatrice Hahn and George Shaw through the AIDS Research and Reference Reagent Program, Division of AIDS, NIAID, NIH.

**pNL4-3**
Proviral full-length, replication and infection competent chimeric DNA of the 5' SmaI-EcoRI fragment of proviral NY5 and the 3' EcoRI-NruI fragment of proviral LAV, which were blunt-end cloned into pUC18 at the PvuII site after removal of polylinker sites. The plasmid was obtained from Dr. Malcolm Martin through the AIDS Research and Reference Reagent Program, Division of AIDS, NIAID, NIH.

**pNL4-3lucR-E-**
Firefly luciferase gene was inserted into the pNL4-3 *nef* gene. Two frameshifts, 5' Env and Vpr amino acid 26, render this clone Env- and Vpr-. The plasmid was obtained from Dr. Nathaniel Landau through the NIH AIDS Research and Reference Reagent Program, Division of AIDS, NIAID, NIH.

**p96 ZM651 gag-opt**
Full-length gag gene of the HIV clone 96ZM651.8 (GenBank accession number AY181195) was artificially reconstructed by substituting original viral codons with those of highly expressed human genes and ligated into the pcDNA3.1(-) expression vector. The gag amino acid sequence is unchanged. Nine base pairs of wildtype viral sequence preceding the initiation codon were retained in this synthetic gene. The size of the translated gag protein is 494 aa. The plasmid was obtained from Drs. Yingying Li, Feng Gao, and Beatrice H. Hahn through the NIH AIDS Research and Reference Reagent Program, Division of AIDS, NIAID, NIH.

**pCAGGS_HIV$_{env}$-NL4-3**
The NL4-3 gp160 envelope was cut out of pNL4-3 as a 3.1kb EcoRI-XhoI fragment and cloned into the pCAGGS vector at the same sites. The plasmid was obtained from Drs. Andrea Marzi and Thomas Gramberg, University Hospital Erlangen, Germany.

**pDOL_HIV$_{env}$-NL4-3**
The NL4-3 gp160 envelope was cut out of pNL4-3 as a 3.1kb SalI-XhoI fragment was introduced into the SalI site of pDOL. pDOL_HIV$_{env}$-NL4-3 contains the open reading frames for the pNL4-3 env, tat, and rev coding regions. Expression is from the Moloney murine virus LTR. The plasmid was obtained from Drs. Eric Freed and Rex Risser through the AIDS Research and Reference Reagent Program, Division of AIDS, NIAID, NIH.

**pSV7d_HIV$_{env}$-ADA**
The SacI-SacI env fragment of the HIV clone ADA were cloned into pSV7d. The gp160 envelope is expressed from an SV40 promoter. No other HIV gene products are expressed. The plasmid was obtained from Drs. Peter Westervelt and John Moore through Drs. Andrea Marzi and Thomas Gramberg, University Hospital Erlangen, Germany.

**pSV7d_HIV$_{env}$-HXB2**
The SacI-XhoI env fragment from pHXB2gpt were cloned into pSV7d. The gp160 envelope is expressed from an SV40 promoter. No other HIV gene products are expressed. The plasmid was obtained from Drs. Kathleen Page and Dan Littman through the AIDS Research and Reference Reagent Program, Division of AIDS, NIAID, NIH.

### 8.4.3. Other Experssion Constructs

**SIV$_{mac}$239 phage**
Originally isolated from a macaque (Mm-239-82) inoculated with cell-free plasma from infected macaques. Virus represents the second successive transmission of virus from macaque Mm-251-79. Infected HUT 78 cells were obtained by inoculation with cell-free serum from Mm-239-82. EcoRI-digested total cell DNA from HUT 78-SIV$_{mac}$239 was inserted into the EcoRI site of λ EMBL4 (Stratagene, Agilent, Waldbronn) and screened for full-length molecular clones. The phage was obtained from Dr. Ronald Desrosiers through the AIDS Research and Reference Reagent Program, Division of AIDS, NIAID, NIH.

**SIV$_{mac}$251 phage**
Splenocytes of a macaque that died of a malignant lymphoma 26 months following inoculation with minced tissue from a spontaneous Macaca mulatta lymphoma were co-cultivated with HUT 78 cells. EcoRI-digested total cell DNA from HUT 78-SIV$_{mac}$251 was inserted into the EcoRI site of λ EMBL4 (Stratagene, Agilent, Waldbronn) and screened for full-length molecular clones. The phage was obtained from Dr. Ronald Desrosiers through the AIDS Research and Reference Reagent Program, Division of AIDS, NIAID, NIH.

**pcDNA3_SIV$_{gp130}$-mac239**
The SIV$_{mac}$239 envelope sequence was PCR amplified and cloned into the pcDNA3 expression vector by using the BamHI and EcoRI sites. The plasmid was obtained from Drs. Andrea Marzi and Stefan Pöhlmann, University Hospital Erlangen, Germany.

**pHEF_VSV$_G$**
The VSV$_G$ envelope sequence was PCR amplified and cloned into the pHEF expression vector. The plasmid was obtained from Dr. Lung-Ji Chang through the AIDS Research and Reference Reagent Program, Division of AIDS, NIAID, NIH.

**pM91.MS.CMV-GFP**
Green fluorescent protein (GFP) gene under control of a CMV promoter was cloned into the expression vector pM91MS by using the NsiI and PacI site, render this clone Env-. pM91MS encodes the complete genome of the amphotropic molecular MLV clone 4070A. The plasmid was obtained from Dr. Carsten Münk, University Hospital Düsseldorf, Germany.

**pHIT60**
Eukaryotic expression vector that contains the MLV gag/pol cassette under the control of the human cytomegalovirus immediate early promoter. The plasmid was obtained from Dr. Karin Metzner, University Zurich, Switzerland.

**pHIT456**
Eukaryotic expression vector that contains the env gene of the amphotropic MLV 4070A under the control of the human cytomegalovirus immediate early promoter. The plasmid was obtained from Dr. Karin Metzner, University Zurich, Switzerland.

**pSV7d_MLV$_{env}$**
Eukaryotic expression vector that contains the env gene of the amphotropic MLV 4070A linked to the MLV LTR. The plasmid was obtained from Drs. Nathaniel Landau and Dan Littman through the AIDS Research and Reference Reagent Program, Division of AIDS, NIAID, NIH.

**pTet-Off**
Expresses the tet-responsive transcriptional activator (tTA) from the strong immediate early promoter of CMV. tTA is a fusion of the tet repressor (TetR) and the negatively charged C-terminal activation domain of the VP16 protein of herpes simplex virus. The pTet-Off vector is used to develop stable Tet-Off cell lines. The plasmid was obtained from Drs. Christian Berens and Wolfgang Hillen, Friedrich-Alexander-University Erlangen-Nuremberg, Germany.

**pTRE2hyg_IRES$_{EMC}$-GFP**
Expression plasmid that expresses a gene of interest from the Tet-responsive minimal CMV promoter lacking the enhancer that is normally part of the complete CMV promoter. The inserted gene of interest will be responsive to the tTA regulatory protein in the Tet-Off system. Consequently, the minimal CMV promoter is silent in the absence of binding of TetR. The vector contains the hygromycin resistance gene as well as a GFP gene under control of the internal ribosome entry site of the encephalomyocarditis virus (IRES$_{EMC}$-GFP). The plasmid was obtained from Dr. Jack T. Stapleton, University of Iowa, Iowa, USA.

## 8.5. Oligonucleotides

### 8.5.1. GBV-C specific Primers and Probes

Sense (5') and anti-sense (3') oligonucleotide primers for cloning of distinct GBV-C proteins and detection of GBV-C RNA were named according the nucleotide sequence of the GBV-C clone AF121950. Start and stop codons are marked by lower case letter in bold. Kozak consensus sequences are underlined and recognition sites of restriction endonucleases are subscribt. Oligonucleotide primer and probes were designed using the Oligo Analysis Tool from Eurofins MWG Operon (Ebersberg) and were purchased from Biomers (Ulm).

| Name | Sequence |
|---|---|
| 5'1(1-20) | TGACGTGGGGGAGTTGATCC |
| 5'GBV-C(96-110) | GGCGACCGGCCAAAA |
| 5'T7 GBV-C(98-110) | TAATACGACTCACTATAGGG..CGACCGGCCAAAA |
| 5'T7tag GBV-C | TAATACGACTCACTATAGGG..CG |
| 5'E1-SP$_{BglII}$ | GCGCGACG$_{AGATCT}$G..CCACCatgGCAGTCCTTCTGC |
| 5'554-573$_{BglII}$ | CGGGAA$_{AGATCTG}$CCAC..CatgGCAGTCCTTCTGCTCC |
| 5'E1-621$_{BglII}$ | CCCCGCACG$_{AGATCT}$..TGTCGAGCGAATGGGCAATATTTC |
| 5'968(968-991) | AAGTGAGTTTTGGAGATGGACTGA |
| 5'981w(981-1003) | AGATGGACTGARCAGYTGGCCTC |
| 5'1164-1190$_{BamHI}$ | GATCGGATCC..GGCGCCCCCGCCTCCGTTTTGGGGTCC |
| 5'1164-1190$_{BglII}$ | GATCAGATCT..GGCGCCCCCGCCTCCGTTTTGGGGTCC |
| 5'1167-1184$_{BamHI}$ | GCA$_{GGATCC}$TGCCACCatg..GCCCCCGCCTCCGTTTTG |
| 5'E2-1167$_{BglII}$ | CGCCCGT$_{AGATCT}$..GCCCCCGCCTCCGTTTTG |
| 5'1193-1218$_{BamHI}$ | GATC$_{GGATC}$..cCCCTTTGACTACGGGTTGAAGTGGC |
| 5'1458w(1457-1477) | YTCCGYGTCTTGGTTTGCCTC |
| 5'1495w(1495-1519) | CGARGATCGATGTGTGGAGTTTGGT |
| 5'1499(1499-1519) | GATCGATGTGTGGAGTTTGGT |
| 5'1516(1495-1516) | CGAAGATCGATGTGTGGAGTTT |
| 5'2319-2340$_{BamHI}$ | GCT$_{GGATCC}$TGCCACCatg..GCCGTGGCGGGTGAAGTTTTTG |
| 5'2478-2498$_{BamHI}$ | GCT$_{GGATCC}$TGCCACCatg..GCTTTCCCGCTGGCACTTTTG |
| 5'3237-3257$_{BglII(2)}$ | TGAGG$_{AGATCT}$GCCACCatg..GCACCAGTTGTCATCCGTC |
| 5'3675w(3675-3697) | CACGCAGTAGGAATGCTSGTGTC |
| 5'5202-5221$_{BamHI}$ | GCA$_{GGATCC}$TGCCACCatg..GACTGGGATGTGAAGGGGGG |
| 5'5835-5857$_{BamHI}$ | GCA$_{GGATCC}$TGCCACCatg..AGCCTTGTCTTCGACTTYATGGC |
| 5'5950(5950-5968) | TGTACTCAGCTAACAACTC |
| 5'6153-6172w$_{BamHI}$ | GCT$_{GGATCC}$TGCCACCatg..GGGTAYGTCTGGGACCTGTG |
| 5'7392-7416$_{BamHI}$ | GCT$_{GGATCC}$TGCCACCatg..TCCTTCTCTTACATTTGGTCTGGGG |
| 5'7868(7868-7888) | CCTGGACTTCCGGATAGCTGA |
| 3'E1-SP$_{BamHI-NotI}$ | TTCTTTT$_{GCGGCCGC}$TTTTTTGGATCC..AGCGTGGGTGGCCGGG |
| 3'GBV-C(163-188) | CTTAAGACCCACCTATAGTGGCTACC |
| 3'GBV lat(261-279) | CTGACGTCGGGCCCTTATT |
| 3'348(330-348) | AAGGGCGACGTGGACCGTA |
| 3'1149-1166$_{NotI}$ | TTTAtta$_{GCGGCCGC}$..GCCTTGCAACATCCCCGC |
| 3'1521(1500-1521) | GCACCAAACTCCACACATCGAT |
| 3'1859w(1839-1858) | TTGGTCATGGYGTAGGACCC |
| 3'2164-2183$_{NotI}$ | CTAG$_{GCGGCCGC}$C..CCAGCGTGGAGGAGGGATGA |
| 3'2225-2244$_{NotI}$ | CTAG$_{GCGGCCGC}$..CCAACCGTGCCTCAGCCAGC |
| 3'2318-2299$_{NotI}$ | CTTTAtta$_{GCGGCCGC}$..AGCGTCCACAGCCGGCAGTC |
| 3'2456-2477$_{MluI}$ | CCTCCG$_{ACGCGT}$TAtta..TCCCCGAGCGAGCTTCCACAAC |
| 3'2456-2477$_{NotI}$ | CTTTAtta$_{GCGGCCGC}$..TCCCCGAGCGAGCTTCCACAAC |
| 3'2456-2477$_{NotI-MluI}$ | TTTAG$_{ACGCG}$taG$_{GCGGCCGC}$..TCCCCGAGCGAGCTTCCACAAC |
| 3'2513(2498-2513) | CGCCGAAATCCCCATC |
| 3'3218-3236$_{MluI}$ | GCCTCCG$_{ACGCGT}$TAtta..AGTCGGGACAAACCCGGGA |
| 3'3218-3236$_{NotI-MluI}$ | TTTAG$_{ACGCGT}$TAG$_{GCGGCCGC}$..AGTCGGGACAAACCCGGGA |
| 3'4547w(4546-4564) | GTWATGGTGGGATCAAGGG |
| 3'5181-5201$_{MluI}$ | GCCTACC$_{ACGCGT}$TAtta..TGTAACCACCACGAGAGACCC |
| 3'5181-5201$_{NotI-MluI}$ | TTTTATG$_{ACGCG}$taG$_{GCGGCCGC}$..TGTAACCACCACGAGAGACCC |
| 3'5816-5834w$_{MluI}$ | CGCCTCCG$_{ACGCGT}$TAtta..AGCMGCATTCACCACGCCC |
| 3'5816-5834w$_{NotI-MluI}$ | TTTAG$_{ACGCGT}$taG$_{GCGGCCGC}$..AGCMGCATTCACCACGCCC |
| 3'6136-6155$_{MluI}$ | GCGGTCCG$_{ACGCGT}$TAtta..CCCCACCTGAACCTCATCCA |
| 3'6136-6155$_{NotI-MluI}$ | TTTTAG$_{ACGCG}$taG$_{GCGGCCGC}$..CCCCACCTGAACCTCATCCA |
| 3'7370-7391w$_{MluI}$ | CGCCTCCG$_{ACGCGT}$TAtta..AGCCAAGGTCTCTTGCCTWGCC |
| 3'7370-7391w$_{NotI-MluI}$ | TTTTAG$_{ACGCG}$taG$_{GCGGCCGC}$..AGCCAAGGTCTCTTGCCTWGCC |
| 3'7410(7393-7410) | ACCARATCTACCAGAAGG |
| 3'8613w(8592-8613) | GGATGATRACCCACCGTGTGAT |
| 3'9062-9080$_{AscI}$ | CT$_{GGGCGCGCC}$TTTAtta..CCCGAAGAGGGCTACGATG |
| 3'9062-9080$_{NotI}$ | TAT$_{GGATCC}$CGC..CCCGAAGAGGGCTACGATG |
| 3'9375(9376-9395) | AGTAGAACCCGGCCTTTGGG |
| 3'9375w(9376-9395) | AGTAGAACCCGGCCTTYGGG |
| GBV-C probe(131-156) | FAM—TGACCGGGATTTACGACCTACCAACCCT—TAMRA |

89

### 8.5.2. Other Gene specific Primer and Probes

Sense (5') and anti-sense (3') primer for cloning and sequencing of different templates were named according the nucleotides of the respective plasmid. Start and stop codons are marked by lower case letter in bold, Kozak consensus sequences are underlined, and recognition sites of restriction endonucleases are subscribed. Oligonucleotide primer and probes were designed using the Oligo Analysis Tool from Eurofins MWG Operon (Ebersberg) and were purchased from Biomers (Ulm).

#### pcDNA3dhfr_E2-TM

| | |
|---|---|
| 5' EPO-SP$_{BglII}$ | GCCCGAGG$_{AGATCT}$GCCACC..**atg**GGGGTGCACGAATGTC |
| 5' E2$_{NotI}$ | ACG$_{GCGGCCGC}$..GATGTCGCAAGGCGCCCCTGC |
| 3' EPO-SP$_{BamHI-NotI}$ | TTCTTTT$_{GCGGCCGC}$TGC$_{GGATCC}$..GTAGTCGCCCAGGACTG |
| 3' E2ΔTM$_{XbaI}$ | CTC$_{TCTAGA}$**tta**..GTTGCCTGCATCCACCTCC |

#### pCEP4_Fc

| | |
|---|---|
| 5' Fc-SP$_{BglII}$ | CGGGCGAGG$_{AGATCT}$..<u>GCCACC</u>**atg**GAGACAG |
| 5' 10414-10392$_{NotI}$ | TA$_{GCGGCCGC}$..CGAACAAAAACTCATCTC |
| 5' 10414-10404$_{BamHI}$ | AATACG$_{GGATCC}$ATA$_{GCGGCCGC}$..CGAACAAAAAC |
| 3' Fc-SP$_{BamHI}$ | TTATTTT$_{GCGGCCGC}$TGC$_G$..$_{GATCC}$ACCAGTGGAACCTG |
| 3' 10371-10353$_{MluI}$ | GCCTACC$_{ACGCGT}$T**Atta**_ATGATGATGATGATGG |
| 3' 10371-10353$_{MluI}$(2) | GCCTACC$_{ACGCGT}$..ATGATGATGATGATGG |

#### pTRE2hyg

| | |
|---|---|
| 5' 37-54 | GTGAAAGTCGAGTTACC |
| 5' 399-418 | TGTTTTGACCTCCATAGAAG |
| 3' 557-540 | CTCACCCTGAAGTTCTCA |
| 3' 721-741 | GAAAATAAGAGGAGACAATGG |
| 3' 983-1000 | CCAGGATGTAGTTGTTTC |

#### pTRE2hyg_IRES$_{EMC}$-GFP_c-myc/His

| | |
|---|---|
| 5' 712-732 | GTTATTTTCCACCATATTGCC |
| 3' 1213-1193 | GGTATTATCATCGTGTTTTC |

#### Adenovirus type 5 (GenBank accession number: X02997)

| | |
|---|---|
| 5' ADP1s(245-269) | GCCGCAGTGGTCTTACATGCACATC |
| 3' AQ1as(376-354) | GCCACGGTGGGGTTTCTAAACTT |
| FAM-ADO(313-285) | FAM—TGCACCAGACCCGGGCTCAGGTACTCCGA—TAMRA |

#### Herpesvirus saimiri (GenBank accession number: GI30348501)

| | |
|---|---|
| 5' HVS(45251-45275) | CTCATTACCAGACCCATGTTATGAA |
| 3' HVS(45357-45334) | CCATTTGCCTGTGTTGAGAGTTAA |
| VIC-HVS(45324-45298) | VIC—CTCCGAGAGAGCCTATCTGAGATGCCC—TAMRA |

### 8.6. Kits and Enzymes

| Kit / Enzyme | Catalog number | Distributor |
|---|---|---|
| AxSYM HIV Ag/Ab Combo | 2G8320 | Abbott Diagnostics, Wiesbaden |
| BigDye Terminator v3.1 | 4337457 | Applied Biosystems, Darmstadt |
| CD19 MicroBeads | 130-050-301 | Miltenyi Biotec, Bergisch Gladbach |
| CD8 MicroBeads | 130-045-201 | Miltenyi Biotec, Bergisch Gladbach |
| CellTiter 96 AQueous One Solution | G3580 | Promega, Mannheim |
| DETACHaBEAD CD4/CD8 | 125.04D | Invitrogen, Groningen |
| DNA free turbo | AM1907 | Applied Biosystems, Darmstadt |

| Kit / Enzyme | Catalog number | Distributor |
|---|---|---|
| Dynal CD4 Positive Isolation Kit | 113.31D | Invitrogen, Groningen |
| Dynal CD8 Positive Isolation Kit | 113.33D | Invitrogen, Groningen |
| Geneclean II | 1001-400 | BIO 101, Carlsbad |
| hCCL3/MIP-1$_{alpha}$ DuoSet ELISA | DY270 | R&D Systems, Wiesbaden |
| hCCL4/MIP-1$_{beta}$ DuoSet ELISA | DY271 | R&D Systems, Wiesbaden |
| hCCL5/RANTES DuoSet ELISA | DY278 | R&D Systems, Wiesbaden |
| hCXCL12/SDF-1 DuoSet ELISA | DY350 | R&D Systems, Wiesbaden |
| High Pure RNA Isolation Kit | 1828665 | Roche Diagnostics, Mannheim |
| High Pure RNA Isolation System | 11828665001 | Roche Diagnostics, Mannheim |
| Human T cell Nucleofector Kit | VPA-1002 | Lonza, Cologne |
| MagNA Pure LC DNA Isolation Kit I | 3310515 | Roche Diagnostics, Mannheim |
| MEGAscript SP6 Kit | AM1330 | Applied Biosystems, Darmstadt |
| MEGAscript SP7 Kit | AM1334 | Applied Biosystems, Darmstadt |
| Murex HIV Antigen mAb | 8E7702 | Abbott Diagnostics, Wiesbaden |
| MycoSensor PCR Assay Kit | 302108 | Agilent, Waldbronn |
| NucleoSpin Plasmid QuickPure | 740615.250 | Macherey-Nagel, Düren |
| Phusion High-Fidelity PCR Kit | F-553 L | New England Biolabs, Frankfurt/M. |
| Platinum Quantitative RT-PCR ThermoScript One-Step | 11731-023 | Invitrogen, Groningen |
| PNGase F | P0704S | New England Biolabs, Frankfurt/M. |
| PureLink HiPure Plasmid Midiprep | K2100-03 | Invitrogen, Groningen |
| PureLink HiPure Plasmid Maxiprep | K2100-06 | Invitrogen, Groningen |
| QIAamp DNA Blood Mini Kit | 51104 | Qiagen, Hilden |
| QIAamp Viral RNA Mini Kit | 52906 | Qiagen, Hilden |
| QIAquick Gel Extraction Kit | 28704 | Qiagen, Hilden |
| QIAquick PCR Purification Kit | 28104 | Qiagen, Hilden |
| QIAshredder | 79654 | Qiagen, Hilden |
| RNeasy Mini Kit | 74104 | Qiagen, Hilden |
| SuperScript III One-Step RT-PCR with Platinum Hifi Taq | 12574-035 | Invitrogen, Groningen |
| SuperScript III Platinum One-Step Quantitative RT-PCR | 11732-020 | Invitrogen, Groningen |
| SuperScript III RNase H- Reverse Transcriptase | 18080-044 | Invitrogen, Groningen |
| TaqMan Universal PCR Master Mix | 4304437 | Applied Biosystems, Darmstadt |
| TOPO TA Cloning Kit with One Shot TOP10 *E. coli* | K4500-01 | Invitrogen, Groningen |
| TOPO XL PCR Cloning Kit with One Shot TOP10 *E. coli* | K4750-10 | Invitrogen, Groningen |
| μ-PLATE Anti-HGVenv | 1822616 | Roche Diagnostics, Mannheim |
| 0.24–9.5 kb RNA ladder | 015620-016 | Invitrogen, Groningen |

## 8.7. Chemicals

| Chemical | Catalog number | Distributor |
|---|---|---|
| 2-Mercaptoethanol | M7522 | Sigma-Aldrich, Taufkirchen |
| Acetic acid | 100063 | Merck, Darmstadt |
| Acetone | 100014 | Merck, Darmstadt |
| Agar | 214010 | Becton Dickinson, Heidelberg |
| Agarose | 15510-027 | Invitrogen, Groningen |
| Ammonium acetate* (5M) | AM9070G | Applied Biosystems, Darmstadt |
| Ammonium chloride | A5666 | Sigma-Aldrich, Taufkirchen |
| Ammonium persulfate (APS) | 101201 | Merck, Darmstadt |
| Amphotericin B | 15290-026 | Invitrogen, Groningen |
| Ampicillin | 11593-027 | Invitrogen, Groningen |
| AmpliTaq DNA Polymerase | N808-0152 | Applied Biosystems, Darmstadt |
| BES | 9134.3 | Carl Roth, Karlsruhe |
| Biocoll (1.077g/ml) | L6115 | Biochrom, Berlin |
| Bromophenol blue | B8026 | Sigma-Aldrich, Taufkirchen |
| BSA | A7030 | Sigma-Aldrich, Taufkirchen |
| BSA, fraction V | A7906 | Sigma-Aldrich, Taufkirchen |
| Citric acid | 100247 | Merck, Darmstadt |
| Coomassie Brilliant Blue G250 | 9598.2 | Carl Roth, Karlsruhe |
| Coomassie Brilliant Blue R250 | 3862.2 | Carl Roth, Karlsruhe |

| Chemical | Catalog number | Distributor |
| --- | --- | --- |
| DABCO | 33480 | Sigma-Aldrich, Taufkirchen |
| dATP, dCTP, dGTP, dTTP set | 1969064 | Roche Diagnostics, Mannheim |
| DCTA | 32869 | Sigma-Aldrich, Taufkirchen |
| Dextran | D4876 | Sigma-Aldrich, Taufkirchen |
| D-Luciferin | 260150 | PJK, Kleinbittersdorf |
| D-Luciferin potassium salt | 82252AS | MoBiTec, Göttingen |
| DMEM | 12100-061 | Invitrogen, Groningen |
| DMSO | 102952 | Merck, Darmstadt |
| Doxycycline hydrochloride | D9891 | Sigma-Aldrich, Taufkirchen |
| DTT | 6908.2 | Carl Roth, Karlsruhe |
| EDTA | 8040.3 | Carl Roth, Karlsruhe |
| EDTA disodium salt dihydrate | E5134 | Sigma-Aldrich, Taufkirchen |
| EDTA* (0.5M, pH 8.0) | AM9260G | Applied Biosystems, Darmstadt |
| EGTA | 3054.3 | Carl Roth, Karlsruhe |
| Ethanol | 100983 | Merck, Darmstadt |
| Ethanol, denatured | K28324108 | Merck, Darmstadt |
| Ethidium bromide | E1510 | Sigma-Aldrich, Taufkirchen |
| Foetal bovine serum (FBS) | P270521 | PAN, Aidenbach |
| G418 | 0239.4 | Carl Roth, Karlsruhe |
| GeneRuler 1kb DNA Ladder Mix | SM0331 | Fermentas, St. Leon-Rot |
| Gentamicin sulfate | 15750-037 | Invitrogen, Groningen |
| Glutardaldehyde | G7776 | Sigma-Aldich, Taufkirchen |
| Glycerol | 15523 | Sigma-Aldich, Taufkirchen |
| Glycine | 104169 | Merck, Darmstadt |
| Guanidinium hydrochloride | 0035.2 | Carl Roth, Karlsruhe |
| Guanidinium thiocyanate | 50990 | Sigma-Aldrich, Taufkirchen |
| HEPES | 9105.4 | Carl Roth, Karlsruhe |
| Hydrochloric acid | 12010 | Sigma-Aldich, Taufkirchen |
| Hydrogen peroxidase | 107209 | Merck, Darmstadt |
| Hygromycin B | CP13.3 | Carl Roth, Karlsruhe |
| Immunostaining pen | MKP-1 | Kisker, Steinfurt |
| Interleukin 2 | 1011456 | Roche Diagnostics, Mannheim |
| Isopropanol | 109624 | Merck, Darmstadt |
| Kanamycin | 11815-032 | Invitrogen, Groningen |
| Lectin | L9132 | Sigma-Aldrich, Taufkirchen |
| L-Glutamine | 21051-024 | Invitrogen, Groningen |
| Lipofectamine 2000 | 11668-019 | Invitrogen, Groningen |
| Lipopolysaccharides from $E.\ coli$ | L-9023 | Sigma-Aldrich, Taufkirchen |
| Magnesium acetate | 1058190250 | Merck, Darmstadt |
| Magnesium chloride | 105833 | Merck, Darmstadt |
| Magnesium chloride* (1M) | AM9530G | Applied Biosystems, Darmstadt |
| Magnesium sulfate | 105886 | Merck, Darmstadt |
| Manganese(II) chloride | 105917 | Merck, Darmstadt |
| MEM | 41500-018 | Invitrogen, Groningen |
| MES | 4256.2 | Carl Roth, Karlsruhe |
| Methanol | 106008 | Merck, Darmstadt |
| Methotrexate hydrate | M8407 | Sigma-Aldrich, Taufkirchen |
| Mowiol 4-88 | 81381 | Sigma-Aldrich, Taufkirchen |
| Neutral Red | N-3246 | Invitrogen, Groningen |
| Ni-NTA agarose beads | 30210 | Qiagen, Hilden |
| Nitric acid | 4989.1 | Carl Roth, Karlsruhe |
| NP-40 | 1754599 | Roche Diagnostics, Mannheim |
| Opti-MemI | 11058021 | Invitrogen, Groningen |
| Orthophosphoric acid | 6366.1 | Carl Roth, Karlsruhe |
| PageRuler prestained Protein Ladder | SM0671 | Fermentas, St. Leon-Rot |
| Panserin 401 | P04-710401 | PAN, Aidenbach |
| Paraformaldehyd | 104005 | Merck, Darmstadt |
| Phytohaemagglutinin | L9132 | Sigma-Aldrich, Taufkirchen |
| PIPES | 9156.2 | Carl Roth, Karlsruhe |

| Chemical | Catalog number | Distributor |
|---|---|---|
| PMSF | 6367.1 | Carl Roth, Karlsruhe |
| Potassium acetate* (3M, pH 5.5) | AM9610 | Applied Biosystems, Darmstadt |
| Potassium bicarbonate | P9144 | Sigma-Aldrich, Taufkirchen |
| Potassium chloride | 104936 | Merck, Darmstadt |
| Potassium chloride* (2M) | AM9640G | Applied Biosystems, Darmstadt |
| Protease inhibitor cocktail | 04693159001 | Roche Diagnostics, Mannheim |
| Puromycin dihydrochloride | 0240.4 | Carl Roth, Karlsruhe |
| rATP | K054.5 | Carl Roth, Karlsruhe |
| RNA storage solution | AM7000 | Applied Biosystems, Darmstadt |
| RNaseOUT rRibonuclease Inhibitor | 10777-019 | Invitrogen, Groningen |
| Roti Imuno-block | T144.1 | Carl Roth, Karlsruhe |
| Roti-Histofix 4% | P087.3 | Carl Roth, Karlsruhe |
| Roti-Nanoquant | K880.1 | Carl Roth, Karlsruhe |
| Rotiphorese GelA (30% Acrylamid) | 3037.1 | Carl Roth, Karlsruhe |
| Rotiphorese GelB (2% Bisacrylamid) | 3039.1 | Carl Roth, Karlsruhe |
| RPMI 1640 | 51800-035 | Invitrogen, Groningen |
| SDS | 2326.2 | Carl Roth, Karlsruhe |
| Sodium chloride | 106404 | Merck, Darmstadt |
| Sodium chloride* (5M) | AM9760G | Applied Biosystems, Darmstadt |
| Sodium hydroxide | 106482 | Merck, Darmstadt |
| Sodium hypochloride | 13440 | Sigma-Aldrich, Taufkirchen |
| Sodium sulfate | 106643 | Merck, Darmstadt |
| Sucrose | S7903 | Sigma-Aldrich, Taufkirchen |
| Sulfuric acid | DY994 | R&D Systems, Wiesbaden |
| TEMED | 2367.1 | Carl Roth, Karlsruhe |
| TRIS | 4855.2 | Carl Roth, Karlsruhe |
| TRIS* (1M, pH 7.0) | AM9850G | Applied Biosystems, Darmstadt |
| TRIS* (1M, pH 8.0) | AM9855G | Applied Biosystems, Darmstadt |
| tri-Sodium citrate dihydrate | 106448 | Merck, Darmstadt |
| TritonX-100 | 3051.2 | Carl Roth, Karlsruhe |
| Trypan blue solution | T8154 | Sigma-Aldrich, Taufkirchen |
| Tween-20 | P1379 | Sigma-Aldrich, Taufkirchen |
| Urea | 666122 | Merck, Darmstadt |
| Water, DEPC treated | AM9915G | Applied Biosystems, Darmstadt |
| Water, pyrogen free | W4502 | Sigma-Aldrich, Taufkirchen |
| Xylene cyanol | X4126 | Sigma-Aldrich, Taufkirchen |

* RNase free

## 8.8. Consumables

| Consumable | Catalog number | Distributor |
|---|---|---|
| Cell culture flask, 25cm$^2$ | 690175 | Sarstedt, Nümbrecht |
| Cell culture flask, 75cm$^2$ | 658175 | Sarstedt, Nümbrecht |
| Cell culture flask, 175cm$^2$ | 660175 | Sarstedt, Nümbrecht |
| Cell culture plate, 6well | 657160 | Greiner Bio-One, Essen |
| Cell culture plate, 12well | 655180 | Greiner Bio-One, Essen |
| Cell culture plate, 24well | 662160 | Greiner Bio-One, Essen |
| Cell culture plate, 96 well flat bottom | 655180 | Greiner Bio-One, Essen |
| Cell culture plate, 96 well round bottom | 650180 | Greiner Bio-One, Essen |
| Cell culture plate, 96 well, white | 3912 | Corning, Schiphol-Rijk |
| Cell scraper | 3010 | Corning, Schiphol-Rijk |
| Cell strainer | 352350 | Becton Dickinson, Heidelberg |
| Centrifugal driven filter unit Centricon, YM-10 | 4241 | Millipore, Schwalbach |
| Centrifugal driven filter unit Centriprep, YM-10 | 4304 | Millipore, Schwalbach |
| Centrifugal driven filter unit Microcon, YM-10 | 42407 | Millipore, Schwalbach |
| Centrifugal driven filter unit Microcon, YM-100 | 42413 | Millipore, Schwalbach |
| Combitip plus, 0.5ml | 30.069.420 | Eppendorf, Hamburg |

| Consumable | Catalog number | Distributor |
|---|---|---|
| Combitip plus, 2.5ml | 30.069.447 | Eppendorf, Hamburg |
| Combitip plus, 5ml | 30.069.455 | Eppendorf, Hamburg |
| Cryo color coder | 375930 | Nunc, Wiesbaden |
| Cryo tube, 1.8ml | 375418 | Nunc, Wiesbaden |
| Cryo tube, 3.6ml | 366524 | Nunc, Wiesbaden |
| Cuvettes 220-1600nm | 30.106.300 | Eppendorf, Hamburg |
| Cuvettes for electroporation, 2mm | 71-2020LE | Peqlab, Erlangen |
| Cuvettes | 67.742 | Sarstedt, Nümbrecht |
| HiTrap Protein G HP | 17040403 | GE Healthcare, Uppsala |
| HiTrap rProtein A FF | 17507901 | GE Healthcare, Uppsala |
| Immuno plate, 96 well | 449824 | Nunc, Wiesbaden |
| Parafilm | PF10 | Hartenstein Laborbedarf, Würzburg |
| PCR microplate sealer | 4311971 | Applied Biosystems, Darmstadt |
| PCR microplate | 4306737 | Applied Biosystems, Darmstadt |
| PCR strip capes | 732-0550 | VWR, Darmstadt |
| PCR strip tubes | 732-0549 | VWR, Darmstadt |
| Pipette tip Safeguard 0.1-10µl | 81-1010 | Peqlab, Erlangen |
| Pipette tip Safeguard 0.5-10µl | 81-1011 | Peqlab, Erlangen |
| Pipette tip Safeguard 0.5-30µl | 81-1020 | Peqlab, Erlangen |
| Pipette tip Safeguard 0.5-200µl | 81-1040 | Peqlab, Erlangen |
| Pipette tip Safeguard 50-1250µl | 81-1060 | Peqlab, Erlangen |
| Pipette tip, 200-1000µl, blue | 2100610 | Ratiolab, Dreieich |
| Pipette tip, 2-200µl, yellow | 70.760.002 | Sarstedt, Nümbrecht |
| Pipette, 5ml | 4051 | Corning, Schiphol-Rijk |
| Pipette, 10ml | 4101 | Corning, Schiphol-Rijk |
| Pipette, 25ml | 4251 | Corning, Schiphol-Rijk |
| PVDF membrane, 0.45µm | IPVH00010 | Millipore, Schwalbach |
| Reaction tube, 1.5ml | 72.690 | Sarstedt, Nümbrecht |
| Reaction tube, 1.5ml | 72.692.005 | Sarstedt, Nümbrecht |
| Reaction tube, 1.5ml* | AM12400 | Applied Biosystems, Darmstadt |
| Reaction tube, 2ml | 72.695 | Sarstedt, Nümbrecht |
| Reaction tube, 5ml | 55.1578 | Sarstedt, Nümbrecht |
| Reaction tube, 15ml | 62.554.502 | Sarstedt, Nümbrecht |
| Reaction tube, 50ml | 62.547.254 | Sarstedt, Nümbrecht |
| Round-bottom tube, 5ml | 352058 | Becton Dickinson, Heidelberg |
| Round-bottom tube, 5ml | 55.1578 | Sarstedt, Nümbrecht |
| Round-bottom tube, 14ml | 187261 | Greiner Bio-One, Essen |
| S-Monovette, 10ml 9NC | 02.1067.001 | Sarstedt, Nümbrecht |
| S-Monovette, 5.5ml LH | 03.1628 | Sarstedt, Nümbrecht |
| S-Monovette, 7.5ml Z | 01.1601 | Sarstedt, Nümbrecht |
| S-Monovette, 9ml K3E | 02.1066.001 | Sarstedt, Nümbrecht |
| Syringe driven filter unit, 0.22µm | P664.1 | Carl Roth, Karlsruhe |
| Syringe, 10ml Luer-lok | 305482 | Becton Dickinson, Heidelberg |
| Syringe, 60ml Luer-lok | 309653 | Becton Dickinson, Heidelberg |
| Vakuum driven filter unit, 500ml, 0.22µm, Stericup | X340.1 | Carl Roth, Karlsruhe |
| Vakuum driven filter unit, 500ml, 0.22µm, Steritop | X336.1 | Carl Roth, Karlsruhe |

* RNase free

# 9. Abbreviations

| | |
|---|---|
| AIDS | Acquired immunodeficiency syndrome |
| APS | Ammonium peroxodisulfat |
| ATP | Adenosin-5'-triphosphate |
| BES | 2-(bis(2-hydroxyethyl)amino)ethanesulfonic acid |
| BSA | Bovine serum albumin |
| CD | Cluster of differentiation |
| DABCO | 1,4-Diazabicyclo(2,2,2)-Octan |
| dATP | 2'-Deoxyadenosine 5'-triphosphate |
| DCTA | 1,2-Diaminocyclohexane tetraacetic acid |
| dCTP | 2'-Deoxycytidine 5'-triphosphate |
| DDM | dodecyl maltoside |
| DEPC | Diethylpyrocarbonate |
| dGTP | 2'-Deoxyguanosine 5'-triphosphate |
| D-Luciferin | D(-)-2-(6'-Hydroxy-benzothiazolyl)D2-thiazoline-4-carboxylic acid |
| DMEM | Dulbecco's modified eagle medium |
| DMSO | Dimethylsulfoxide |
| DNA | Deoxyribonucleic acid |
| Doxy | Doxycycline hydrochloride |
| DTT | 1,4-Dithiothreit |
| dTTP | 2'-Deoxythymidine 5'-triphosphate |
| EDTA | Ethylene diamine tetraacetic acid |
| EGTA | Ethylene glycol tetraacetic acid |
| EtBr | Ethidium bromide |
| FBS | Foetal bovine serum |
| FITC | Fluorescein isothiocyanate |
| G418 | Geneticin disulfate |
| HEPES | 4-(2-Hydroxyethyl)-1-piperazineethanesulfonic acid |
| HIS | Histidine |
| HIV | Human immunodeficiency virus |
| HRP | Horseradish peroxidase |
| HVS | *Herpesvirus saimiri* |
| Imidazole | 1,3-Diaza-2,4-cyclopentadiene |
| MES | 2-(N-Morpholino)ethanesulfonic acid |
| MIP | Macrophage inflammatory protein |
| MOPS | 3-(N-Morpholino)propanesulfonic acid |
| Ni-NTA | Nickel-nitrilotriacetic acid |
| NP-40 | Nonidet P-40, Octylphenolpoly(ethylenglycolether) |
| ORF | Open reading frame |
| PE | Phycoerythrin |
| PEG | Polyethylene glycol |
| PFA | Paraformaldehyde |
| PIPES | Piperazin-1,4-bis(2-ethansulfonic acid) |
| PMSF | Phenylmethanesulphonylfluoride |
| PNGase F | N-Glycosidase F |
| PVDF | Polyvinylidene fluoride |
| RANTES | Regulated upon activation normal T cell expressed and secreted |
| RNA | Ribonucleic acid |
| RPMI | Roswell park memorial institute |
| SDF | Stomal cell-derived factor |
| SDS | Sodiumdodecyl sulfate |
| ß-ME | 2- Mercaptoethanol |
| TCEP | Tris (2-carboxylethyl) phosphine hydrochloride |
| TEMED | Tetramethylethane-1,2-diamine |
| TFMS | Trifluoromethanesulfonic |
| Tris | 1-[bis(2,3-dibromopropoxy)phosphoryloxy]-2,3-dipromo-propane |
| Tween-20 | Polyoxyethylenesorbitan monolaurate |

# 10. Bibliography

[1] Abbott Laboratories. Reverenz an Prof. F. Deinhardt. (1996).

[2] Akbar,N. *et al.* The prevalence of GB virus C, risk factors and its relationship with other hepatitis viruses in a general population in Jakarta, Indonesia. *Hepatology Research* 13, 193-204 (1999).

[3] Alam,S.M. *et al.* The role of antibody polyspecificity and lipid reactivity in binding of broadly neutralizing anti-HIV-1 envelope human monoclonal antibodies 2F5 and 4E10 to glycoprotein 41 membrane proximal envelope epitopes. *J Immunol* 178, 4424-4435 (2007).

[4] Alam,S.M. *et al.* Role of HIV membrane in neutralization by two broadly neutralizing antibodies. *Proc Natl Acad Sci USA* 106, 20234-20239 (2009).

[5] Ali,N., Tardif,K.D. & Siddiqui,A. Cell-free replication of the hepatitis C virus subgenomic replicon. *J Virol* 76, 12001-12007 (2002).

[6] Aloia,R.C., Tian,H. & Jensen,F.C. Lipid composition and fluidity of the human immunodeficiency virus envelope and host cell plasma membranes. *Proc Natl Acad Sci USA* 90, 5181-5185 (1993).

[7] Alter,H.J. *et al.* The incidence of transfusion-associated hepatitis G virus infection and its relation to liver disease. *N Engl J Med* 336, 747-754 (1997).

[8] Alter,H.J. *et al.* Detection of antibody to hepatitis C virus in prospectively followed transfusion recipients with acute and chronic non-A, non-B hepatitis. *N Engl J Med* 321, 1494-1500 (1989).

[9] Alter,M.J. *et al.* The natural history of community-acquired hepatitis C in the United States. The Sentinel Counties Chronic non-A, non-B Hepatitis Study Team. *N Engl J Med* 327, 1899-1905 (1992).

[10] Amara,A. *et al.* HIV coreceptor downregulation as antiviral principle: SDF-1alpha-dependent internalization of the chemokine receptor CXCR4 contributes to inhibition of HIV replication. *J Exp Med* 186, 139-146 (1997).

[11] Ansari,A.W., Heiken,H., Moenkemeyer,M. & Schmidt,R.E. Dichotomous effects of C-C chemokines in HIV-1 pathogenesis. *Immunol Lett* 110, 1-5 (2007).

[12] Asada,H., Klaus-Kovtun,V., Golding,H., Katz,S.I. & Blauvelt,A. Human herpesvirus 6 infects dendritic cells and suppresses HIV-1 replication in coinfected cultures. *J Virol* 73, 4019-4028 (1999).

[13] Bae,H.G., Nitsche,A., Teichmann,A., Biel,S.S. & Niedrig,M. Detection of yellow fever virus: a comparison of quantitative real-time PCR and plaque assay. *J Virol Methods* 110, 185-191 (2003).

[14] Barre-Sinoussi,F. *et al.* Isolation of a T-lymphotropic retrovirus from a patient at risk for acquired immune deficiency syndrome (AIDS). *Science* 220, 868-871 (1983).

[15] Barrero-Villar,M. *et al.* PI4P5-kinase Ialpha is required for efficient HIV-1 entry and infection of T cells. *J Immunol* 181, 6882-6888 (2008).

[16] Bartosch,B. & Cosset,F.L. Cell entry of hepatitis C virus. *Virology* 348, 1-12 (2006).

[17] Belshe,R.B. *et al.* Safety and immunogenicity of a fully glycosylated recombinant gp160 human immunodeficiency virus type 1 vaccine in subjects at low risk of infection. *J Infect Dis* 168, 1387-1395 (1993).

[18] Belyaev,A.S. *et al.* Hepatitis G virus encodes protease activities which can effect processing of the virus putative nonstructural proteins. *J Virol* 72, 868-872 (1998).

[19] Belz,G.T. & Masson,F. Interleukin-2 tickles T cell memory. *Immunity* 32, 7-9 (2010).

[20] Berkhout,B. *et al.* Characterization of the anti-HIV effects of native lactoferrin and other milk proteins and protein-derived peptides. *Antiviral Res* 55, 341-355 (2002).

[21] Berkowitz,R.D. & Goff,S.P. Point mutations in Moloney murine leukemia virus envelope protein: effects on infectivity, virion association, and superinfection resistance. *Virology* 196, 748-757 (1993).

[22] Berzsenyi,M.D., Bowden,D.S. & Roberts,S.K. GB virus C: Insights into co-infection. *J Clin Virol* 33, 257-266 (2005).

[23] Biesinger,B. *et al.* Stable growth transformation of human T lymphocytes by herpesvirus saimiri. *Proc Natl Acad Sci USA* 89, 3116-3119 (1992).

[24] Birk,M., Lindback,S. & Lidman,C. No influence of GB virus C replication on the prognosis in a cohort of HIV-1-infected patients. *AIDS* 16, 2482-2485 (2002).

[25] Birkmann,A. *et al.* Cell surface heparan sulfate is a receptor for human herpesvirus 8 and interacts with envelope glycoprotein K8.1. *J Virol* 75, 11583-11593 (2001).

[26] Bitonti,A.J. *et al.* Pulmonary delivery of an erythropoietin Fc fusion protein in non-human primates through an immunoglobulin transport pathway. *Proc Natl Acad Sci USA* 101, 9763-9768 (2004).

[27] Bjorkman,P. *et al.* GB virus C during the natural course of HIV-1 infection: viremia at diagnosis does not predict mortality. *AIDS* 18, 877-886 (2004).

[28] Bjorkman,P. *et al.* GB virus C/hepatitis G virus infection in patients investigated for chronic liver disease and in the general population in southern Sweden. *Scand J Infect Dis* 33, 611-617 (2001).

[29] Blackard,J.T. & Sherman,K.E. HCV/HIV co-infection: time to re-evaluate the role of HIV in the liver? *J Viral Hepat* 15, 323-330 (2008).

[30] Blair,C.S. *et al.* Prevalence, incidence, and clinical characteristics of hepatitis G virus/GB virus C infection in Scottish blood donors. *J Infect Dis* 178, 1779-1782 (1998).

[31] Borgia,G., Reynaud,L., Gentile,I. & Piazza,M. HIV and hepatitis C virus: facts and controversies. *Infection* 31, 232-240 (2003).

[32] Borrow,P., Lewicki,H., Hahn,B.H., Shaw,G.M. & Oldstone,M.B. Virus-specific CD8+ cytotoxic T-lymphocyte activity associated with control of viremia in primary human immunodeficiency virus type 1 infection. *J Virol* 68, 6103-6110 (1994).

[33] Boyd,M.A. Improvements in antiretroviral therapy outcomes over calendar time. *Curr Opin HIV AIDS* 4, 194-199 (2009).

[34] Boyer,J.D. *et al.* Vaccination of seronegative volunteers with a human immunodeficiency virus type 1 env/rev DNA vaccine induces antigen-specific proliferation and lymphocyte production of beta-chemokines. *J Infect Dis* 181, 476-483 (2000).

[35] Brenchley,J.M. *et al.* CD4+ T cell depletion during all stages of HIV disease occurs predominantly in the gastrointestinal tract. *J Exp Med* 200, 749-759 (2004).

[36] Brown,B.K. *et al.* Monoclonal antibodies to phosphatidylinositol phosphate neutralize human immunodeficiency virus type 1: role of phosphate-binding subsites. *J Virol* 81, 2087-2091 (2007).

[37] Brugger,B. *et al.* The HIV lipidome: a raft with an unusual composition. *Proc Natl Acad Sci USA* 103, 2641-2646 (2006).

[38] Brumme,Z.L. *et al.* No association between GB virus-C viremia and virological or immunological failure after starting initial antiretroviral therapy. *AIDS* 16, 1929-1933 (2002).

[39] Busch,M.P. *et al.* Factors influencing human immunodeficiency virus type 1 transmission by blood transfusion. Transfusion Safety Study Group. *J Infect Dis* 174, 26-33 (1996).

[40] Camaur,D. & Trono,D. Characterization of HIV-1 Vif particle incorporation. *J Virol* 70, 6106-6111 (1996).

[41] Caputo,A. et al. HIV-1 Tat-based vaccines: an overview and perspectives in the field of HIV/AIDS vaccine development. *Int Rev Immunol* 28, 285-334 (2009).

[42] CDC. Pneumocystis pneumonia - Los Angeles. *MMWR Morb Mortal Wkly Rep.* 30, 1-3 (1981).

[43] CDC. Epidemiologic Notes and Reports Pneumocystis carinii Pneumonia among Persons with Hemophilia A. *MMWR Morb Mortal Wkly Rep.* 31, 365-367 (1982).

[44] Chan,R. et al. Retroviruses, human immunodeficiency virus and murine leukemia virus are enriched in phosphoinositides. *J Virol* 82, 11228-11238 (2008).

[45] Chaurio,R.A. et al. Phospholipids: key players in apoptosis and immune regulation. *Molecules* 14, 4892-4914 (2009).

[46] Chen,R., Quinones-Mateu,M.E. & Mansky,L.M. Drug resistance, virus fitness and HIV-1 mutagenesis. *Curr Pharm Des* 10, 4065-4070 (2004).

[47] Chen,Z. et al. GB virus B disrupts RIG-I signaling by NS3/4A-mediated cleavage of the adaptor protein MAVS. *J Virol* 81, 964-976 (2007).

[48] Choe,H. et al. The beta-chemokine receptors CCR3 and CCR5 facilitate infection by primary HIV-1 isolates. *Cell* 85, 1135-1148 (1996).

[49] Choo,Q.L. et al. Isolation of a cDNA clone derived from a blood-borne non-A, non-B viral hepatitis genome. *Science* 244, 359-362 (1989).

[50] Christensen,P.B. et al. GB virus C epidemiology in Denmark: different routes of transmission in children and low- and high-risk adults. *J Med Virol* 70, 156-162 (2003).

[51] Chukkapalli,V., Hogue,I.B., Boyko,V., Hu,W.S. & Ono,A. Interaction between the human immunodeficiency virus type 1 Gag matrix domain and phosphatidylinositol-(4,5)-bisphosphate is essential for efficient gag membrane binding. *J Virol* 82, 2405-2417 (2008).

[52] Claret,G. et al. The prevalence of GB virus C/hepatitis G virus RNA among healthy and HCV-infected Catalan children. *Eur J Pediatr.* 167, 991-994 (2008).

[53] Clavel,F. et al. Isolation of a new human retrovirus from West African patients with AIDS. *Science* 233, 343-346 (1986).

[54] Cocchi,F. et al. Identification of RANTES, MIP-1 alpha, and MIP-1 beta as the major HIV-suppressive factors produced by CD8+ T cells. *Science* 270, 1811-1815 (1995).

[55] Coffin,J. et al. HIV. *Science* 232, 697 (1986).

[56] Cohen,E.A., Subbramanian,R.A. & Gottlinger,H.G. Role of auxiliary proteins in retroviral morphogenesis. *Curr Top Microbiol Immunol* 214, 219-235 (1996).

[57] Compston,L.I. et al. Prevalence of persistent and latent viruses in untreated patients infected with HIV-1 from Ghana, West Africa. *J Med Virol* 81, 1860-1868 (2009).

[58] Connor,R.I., Chen,B.K., Choe,S. & Landau,N.R. Vpr is required for efficient replication of human immunodeficiency virus type-1 in mononuclear phagocytes. *Virology* 206, 935-944 (1995).

[59] Cuceanu,N.M., Tuplin,A. & Simmonds,P. Evolutionarily conserved RNA secondary structures in coding and non-coding sequences at the 3' end of the hepatitis G virus/GB-virus C genome. *J Gen Virol* 82, 713-722 (2001).

[60] Cullen,B.R. & Greene,W.C. Functions of the auxiliary gene products of the HIV type 1. *Virology* 178, 1-5 (1990).

[61] Cunningham,A.L., Carbone,F. & Geijtenbeek,T.B. Langerhans cells and viral immunity. *Eur J Immunol* 38, 2377-2385 (2008).

[62] D'Arena,G. et al. Flow cytometric characterization of human umbilical cord blood lymphocytes: immunophenotypic features. *Haematologica* 83, 197-203 (1998).

[63] Daniel,M.D. et al. Simian immunodeficiency virus from African green monkeys. *J Virol* 62, 4123-4128 (1988).

[64] Danta,M. & Dusheiko,G.M. Acute HCV in HIV-positive individuals - a review. *Curr Pharm Des* 14, 1690-1697 (2008).

[65] Dau,B. & Holodniy,M. Novel targets for antiretroviral therapy: clinical progress to date. *Drugs* 69, 31-50 (2009).

[66] Dawson,G.J. et al. Prevalence studies of GB virus-C infection using reverse transcriptase-polymerase chain reaction. *J Med Virol* 50, 97-103 (1996).

[67] De Renzo,A. et al. High prevalence of hepatitis G virus infection in Hodgkin's disease and B-cell lymphoproliferative disorders: absence of correlation with hepatitis C virus infection. *Haematologica* 87, 714-718 (2002).

[68] Deinhardt,F., Holmes,A.W., Capps,R.B. & Popper,H. Studies on the transmission of human viral hepatitis to marmoset monkeys. I. Transmission of disease, serial passages, and description of liver lesions. *J Exp Med* 125, 673-688 (1967).

[69] Deinhardt,F., Peterson,D., Cross,G., Wolfe,L & Holmes,A.W. Hepatitis in marmosets. *Am J Med Sci* 270, 73-80 (1975).

[70] Demmel,L. et al. The clathrin adaptor Gga2p is a phosphatidylinositol 4-phosphate effector at the Golgi exit. *Mol Biol Cell* 19, 1991-2002 (2008).

[71] Deng,H. et al. Identification of a major co-receptor for primary isolates of HIV-1. *Nature* 381, 661-666 (1996).

[72] Dille,B.J. et al. An ELISA for detection of antibodies to the E2 protein of GB virus C. *J Infect Dis* 175, 458-461 (1997).

[73] Duh,E.J., Maury,W.J., Folks,T.M., Fauci,A.S. & Rabson,A.B. Tumor necrosis factor alpha activates HIV-1 through induction of nuclear factor binding to the NF-kappa B sites in the long terminal repeat. *Proc Natl Acad Sci USA* 86, 5974-5978 (1989).

[74] Dumont,J.A., Low,S.C., Peters,R.T. & Bitonti,A.J. Monomeric Fc fusions: impact on pharmacokinetic and biological activity of protein therapeutics. *BioDrugs* 20, 151-160 (2006).

[75] Dunfee,R. et al. Mechanisms of HIV-1 neurotropism. *Curr HIV Res* 4, 267-278 (2006).

[76] Earl,P.L., Doms,R.W. & Moss,B. Oligomeric structure of the HIV-1 envelope glycoprotein. *Proc Natl Acad Sci USA* 87, 648-652 (1990).

[77] Egger,D. et al. Expression of hepatitis C virus proteins induces distinct membrane alterations including a candidate viral replication complex. *J Virol* 76, 5974-5984 (2002).

[78] England,K., Thorne,C. & Newell,M.L. Vertically acquired paediatric coinfection with HIV and hepatitis C virus. *Lancet Infect Dis* 6, 83-90 (2006).

[79] Feinberg,M.B., Jarrett,R.F., Aldovini,A., Gallo,R.C. & Wong-Staal,F. HTLV-III expression and production involve complex regulation at the levels of splicing and translation of viral RNA. *Cell* 46, 807-817 (1986).

[80] Feng,Y., Broder,C.C., Kennedy,P.E. & Berger,E.A. HIV-1 entry cofactor: functional cDNA cloning of a seven-transmembrane, G protein-coupled receptor. *Science* 272, 872-877 (1996).

[81] Ferron,F., Bussetta,C., Dutartre,H. & Canard,B. The modeled structure of the RNA dependent RNA polymerase of GBV-C Virus suggests a role for motif E in Flaviviridae RNA polymerases. *BMC Bioinformatics* 6, 255 (2005).

[82] Feucht,H.H. et al. GB virus C infection and liver transplantation: increased risk of transfusion-transmitted infection. *Blood* 89, 2223-2224 (1997).

[83] Feucht,H.H., Zollner,B., Polywka,S. & Laufs,R. Vertical transmission of hepatitis G. *Lancet* 347, 615-616 (1996).

[84] Fickenscher,H. & Fleckenstein,B. Herpesvirus saimiri. *Philos Trans R Soc Lond B Biol Sci* 356, 545-567 (2001).

[85] Fischer,M.J. et al. Hepatitis C and the risk of kidney disease and mortality in veterans with HIV. *J Acquir Immune Defic Syndr* 53, 222-226 (2010).

[86] Flint,S.J., Enquist,L.W., Racaniello,V.R. & Skalka,A.M. Principles of Virology. Book (2004).

[87] Fogeda,M. et al. Existence of distinct GB virus C/hepatitis G virus variants with different tropism. *J Virol* 74, 7936-7942 (2000).

[88] Fogeda,M. et al. In vitro infection of human peripheral blood mononuclear cells by GB virus C/Hepatitis G virus. *J Virol* 73, 4052-4061 (1999).

[89] Forns,X. et al. Hepatitis G virus infection in a haemodialysis unit: prevalence and clinical implications. *Nephrol Dial Transplant* 12, 956-960 (1997).

[90] Freed,E.O. HIV-1 replication. *Somat Cell Mol Genet* 26, 13-33 (2001).

[91] Frey,S.E. et al. Evidence for probable sexual transmission of the hepatitis g virus. *Clin Infect Dis* 34, 1033-1038 (2002).

[92] Frost,S.D. et al. Neutralizing antibody responses drive the evolution of human immunodeficiency virus type 1 envelope during recent HIV infection. *Proc Natl Acad Sci USA* 102, 18514-18519 (2005).

[93] Gahery-Segard,H. et al. Multiepitopic B- and T-cell responses induced in humans by a human immunodeficiency virus type 1 lipopeptide vaccine. *J Virol* 74, 1694-1703 (2000).

[94] Gallo,R.C. et al. Isolation of human T-cell leukemia virus in acquired immune deficiency syndrome (AIDS). *Science* 220, 865-867 (1983).

[95] Gamberini,M.R. et al. HCV and HGV infection, iron overload and liver disease in multitransfused patients with thalassaemia and persistently normal or abnormal transaminase levels. *Pediatr. Endocrinol Rev* 2 Suppl 2, 259-266 (2004).

[96] Gao,F. et al. Human infection by genetically diverse SIVSM-related HIV-2 in west Africa. *Nature* 358, 495-499 (1992).

[97] Gasper-Smith,N. et al. Induction of plasma (TRAIL), TNFR-2, Fas ligand, and plasma microparticles after human immunodeficiency virus type 1 (HIV-1) transmission: implications for HIV-1 vaccine design. *J Virol* 82, 7700-7710 (2008).

[98] Gelderblom,H.R., Hausmann,E.H., Ozel,M., Pauli,G. & Koch,M.A. Fine structure of HIV and immunolocalization of structural proteins. *Virology* 156, 171-176 (1987).

[99] Gelderblom,H.R., Ozel,M. & Pauli,G. Morphogenesis and morphology of HIV. Structure-function relations. *Arch Virol* 106, 1-13 (1989).

[100] Geonnotti AR et al. Endotoxin-mediated inhibition of Human Immunodeficiency Virus Type 1: a cautionary note for neutralizing antibody assays. *16th Conference of retroviruses and opportunistic infections*, Abstract 328b (2009).

[101] George,S.L., Varmaz,D. & Stapleton,J.T. GB Virus C Replicates in Primary T and B Lymphocytes. *J Infect Dis* 193, 451-454 (2006).

[102] George,S.L., Xiang,J. & Stapleton,J.T. Clinical isolates of GB virus type C vary in their ability to persist and replicate in peripheral blood mononuclear cell cultures. *Virology* 316, 191-201 (2003).

[103] Gomez,C. & Hope,T.J. The ins and outs of HIV replication. *Cell Microbiol* 7, 621-626 (2005).

[104] Gonda,M.A. et al. Sequence homology and morphologic similarity of HTLV-III and visna virus, a pathogenic lentivirus. *Science* 227, 173-177 (1985).

[105] Gorry,P.R., Churchill,M., Crowe,S.M., Cunningham,A.L. & Gabuzda,D. Pathogenesis of macrophage tropic HIV-1. *Curr HIV Res* 3, 53-60 (2005).

[106] Gossen,M. & Bujard,H. Tight control of gene expression in mammalian cells by tetracycline-responsive promoters. *Proc Natl Acad Sci USA* 89, 5547-5551 (1992).

[107] Gossen,M. et al. Transcriptional activation by tetracyclines in mammalian cells. *Science* 268, 1766-1769 (1995).

[108] Greene,W.C. & Peterlin,B.M. Charting HIV's remarkable voyage through the cell: Basic science as a passport to future therapy. *Nat Med* 8, 673-680 (2002).

[109] Grivel,J.C. et al. Suppression of CCR5- but not CXCR4-tropic HIV-1 in lymphoid tissue by human herpesvirus 6. *Nat Med* 7, 1232-1235 (2001).

[110] Grivel,J.C. et al. Pathogenic effects of human herpesvirus 6 in human lymphoid tissue ex vivo. *J Virol* 77, 8280-8289 (2003).

[111] Gutierrez,R.A. et al. Seroprevalence of GB virus C and persistence of RNA and antibody. *J Med Virol* 53, 167-173 (1997).

[112] Hall,H.I. et al. Estimation of HIV incidence in the United States. *JAMA* 300, 520-529 (2008).

[113] Hallenberger,S. et al. Inhibition of furin-mediated cleavage activation of HIV-1 glycoprotein gp160. *Nature* 360, 358-361 (1992).

[114] Harada,H. et al. Development of cell systems to study viral gene transcription at the initial phase of Epstein-Barr virus infection. *Virus Genes* 1, 73-82 (1987).

[115] Hartley,O., Klasse,P.J., Sattentau,Q.J. & Moore,J.P. V3: HIV's switch-hitter. *AIDS Res Hum Retroviruses* 21, 171-189 (2005).

[116] Hassoba,H.M. et al. Antibody to GBV-C second envelope glycoprotein (anti-GBV-C E2): is it a marker for immunity? *J Med Virol* 53, 354-360 (1997).

[117] Haste,A.P., Nielsen,M. & Lund,O. Prediction of residues in discontinuous B-cell epitopes using protein 3D structures. *Protein Sci* 15, 2558-2567 (2006).

[118] He,J. et al. Human immunodeficiency virus type 1 viral protein R (Vpr) arrests cells in the G2 phase of the cell cycle by inhibiting p34cdc2 activity. *J Virol* 69, 6705-6711 (1995).

[119] Heeney,J.L. et al. A vaccine strategy utilizing a combination of three different chimeric vectors which share specific vaccine antigens. *J Med Primatol.* 29, 268-273 (2000).

[120] Heringlake,S. et al. GB virus C/hepatitis G virus infection: a favorable prognostic factor in human immunodeficiency virus-infected patients? *J Infect Dis* 177, 1723-1726 (1998).

[121] Heringlake,S. et al. GBV-C/HGV is not the major cause of autoimmune hepatitis. *Hepatology* 25, 980-984 (1996).

[122] Herrera,E., Gomara,M.J., Mazzini,S., Ragg,E. & Haro,I. Synthetic peptides of hepatitis G virus (GBV-C/HGV) in the selection of putative peptide inhibitors of the HIV-1 fusion peptide. *J Phys Chem B* 113, 7383-7391 (2009).

[123] Herrero,M.D., Rivas,P., Rallon,N.I., Ramirez-Olivencia,G. & Puente,S. HIV and malaria. *AIDS Rev* 9, 88-98 (2007).

[124] Hirsch,V.M., Olmsted,R.A., Murphey-Corb,M., Purcell,R.H. & Johnson,P.R. An African primate lentivirus (SIVsm) closely related to HIV-2. *Nature* 339, 389-392 (1989).

[125] Huang,C. Receptor-Fc fusion therapeutics, traps, and MIMETIBODY technology. *Curr Opin Biotechnol* 20, 692-699 (2009).

[126] Huang,L & Crothers,K. HIV-associated opportunistic pneumonias. *Respirology* 14, 474-485 (2009).

[127] Huet,T., Cheynier,R., Meyerhans,A., Roelants,G. & Wain-Hobson,S. Genetic organization of a chimpanzee lentivirus related to HIV-1. *Nature* 345, 356-359 (1990).

[128] Hupfeld,J. & Efferth,T. Review. Drug resistance of HIV and overcoming it by natural products. *In Vivo* 23, 1-6 (2009).

[129] Jung,S. GBV-C spezifische Inhibition der Replikation Humaner Immundefizienz-Viren. Diploma thesis (2004).

[130] Jung,S. et al. HIV entry inhibition by the envelope 2 glycoprotein of GB virus C. *AIDS* 21, 645-647 (2007).

[131] Jung,S. et al. Inhibition of HIV strains by GB virus C in cell culture can be mediated by CD4 and CD8 T-lymphocyte derived soluble factors. *AIDS* 19, 1267-1272 (2005).

[132] Kallinowski,B. *et al.* Clinical impact of HGV infection in heart and liver transplant recipients. *Transplant Proc* 34, 2288-2291 (2002).

[133] Kanda,T. *et al.* GB virus-C RNA in Japanese patients with hepatocellular carcinoma and cirrhosis. *Hepatology* 27, 464-469 (1997).

[134] Kao,J.H. *et al.* Interspousal transmission of GB virus-C/hepatitis G virus: a comparison with hepatitis C virus. *J Med Virol* 53, 348-353 (1997).

[135] Kapoor,S., Gupta,R.K., Das,B.C. & Kar,P. Clinical implications of hepatitis G virus (HGV) infection in patients of acute viral hepatitis & fulminant hepatic failure. *Indian J Med Res* 112, 121-127 (2000).

[136] Kashuba,A.D. *et al.* Antiretroviral-drug concentrations in semen: implications for sexual transmission of human immunodeficiency virus type 1. *Antimicrob Agents Chemother* 43, 1817-1826 (1999).

[137] Kato,T. *et al.* Amino acid substitutions in NS5A region of GB virus C and response to interferon therapy. *J Med Virol* 57, 376-382 (1999).

[138] Kaufman,T.M., McLinden,J.H., Xiang,J., Engel,A.M. & Stapleton,J.T. The GBV-C envelope glycoprotein E2 does not interact specifically with CD81. *AIDS* 21, 1045-1048 (2007).

[139] Keck,Z.Y. *et al.* Mutations in hepatitis C virus E2 located outside the CD81 binding sites lead to escape from broadly neutralizing antibodies but compromise virus infectivity. *J Virol* 83, 6149-6160 (2009).

[140] Keck,Z.Y. *et al.* A point mutation leading to hepatitis C virus escape from neutralization by a monoclonal antibody to a conserved conformational epitope. *J Virol* 82, 6067-6072 (2008).

[141] Keefer,M.C. *et al.* Safety and immunogenicity of Env 2-3, a HIV-1 candidate vaccine, in combination with a novel adjuvant, MTP-PE/MF59. NIAID AIDS Vaccine Evaluation Group. *AIDS Res Hum Retroviruses* 12, 683-693 (1996).

[142] Kiertiburanakul,S. & Sungkanuparph,S. Emerging of HIV drug resistance: epidemiology, diagnosis, treatment and prevention. *Curr HIV Res* 7, 273-278 (2009).

[143] Kikukawa,R. *et al.* Differential susceptibility to the acquired immunodeficiency syndrome retrovirus in cloned cells of human leukemic T-cell line Molt-4. *J Virol* 57, 1159-1162 (1986).

[144] Kilmarx,P.H. Global epidemiology of HIV. *Curr Opin HIV AIDS* 4, 240-246 (2009).

[145] Kim,J.P. & Fry,K.E. Molecular characterization of the hepatitis G virus. *J Viral Hepat* 4, 77-79 (1997).

[146] Kleinman,S. Hepatitis G virus biology, epidemiology, and clinical manifestations: Implications for blood safety. *Transfus Med Rev* 15, 201-212 (2001).

[147] Kohn,G., Mellman,W.J., Moorhead,P.S., Loftus,J. & Henle,G. Involvement of C group chromosomes in five Burkitt lymphoma cell lines. *J Natl Cancer Inst.* 38, 209-222 (1967).

[148] Kondo,Y. *et al.* Analysis of conserved ambisense sequences within GB virus C. *J Infect Dis* 178, 1185-1188 (1998).

[149] Koup,R.A. *et al.* Temporal association of cellular immune responses with the initial control of viremia in primary HIV type 1 syndrome. *J Virol* 68, 4650-4655 (1994).

[150] Kovacs,J.A. *et al.* Induction of humoral and cell-mediated anti-HIV responses in HIV sero-negative volunteers by immunization with recombinant gp160. *J Clin Invest* 92, 919-928 (1993).

[151] Krajden,M. *et al.* GBV-C/hepatitis G virus infection and non-Hodgkin lymphoma: a case control study. *Int J Cancer* (2009).

[152] Kuznetsov,Y.G., Victoria,J.G., Robinson,W.E., Jr. & McPherson,A. Atomic force microscopy investigation of HIV and HIV-infected lymphocytes. *J Virol* 77, 11896-11909 (2003).

[153] Laemmli,U.K. Cleavage of structural proteins during the assembly of the head of bacteriophage T4. *Nature* 227, 680-685 (1970).

[154] Larsen,J.E., Lund,O. & Nielsen,M. Improved method for predicting linear B-cell epitopes. *Immunome Res* 2, 2 (2006).

[155] Laskus,T., Radkowski,M., Wang,L.F., Vargas,H. & Rakela,J. Lack of evidence for hepatitis G virus replication in the livers of patients coinfected with hepatitis C and G viruses. *J Virol* 71, 7804-7806 (1997).

[156] Le Rouzic,E. & Benichou,S. The Vpr protein from HIV-1: distinct roles along the viral life cycle. *Retrovirology* 2, 11 (2005).

[157] Leary,T.P. *et al.* Sequence and genomic organization of GBV-C: a novel member of the flaviviridae associated with human non-A-E hepatitis. *J Med Virol* 48, 60-67 (1996).

[158] Lefrere,J.J. *et al.* Carriage of GB virus C/hepatitis G virus RNA is associated with a slower immunologic, virologic, and clinical progression of human immunodeficiency virus disease in coinfected persons. *J Infect Dis* 179, 783-789 (1999).

[159] Lefrere,J.J. *et al.* High rate of GB virus type C/HGV transmission from mother to infant: possible implications for the prevalence of infection in blood donors. *Transfusion* 40, 602-607 (2000).

[160] Lei,X., Yoshihiro,A., Liu,L. & Zhao,L. GB virus-C infection in Chinese patients with hepatocellular carcinoma. *Hua Xi Yi Ke Da Xue Xue Bao* 30, 431-433 (1999).

[161] Letourneau,S., Krieg,C., Pantaleo,G. & Boyman,O. IL-2- and CD25-dependent immunoregulatory mechanisms in the homeostasis of T-cell subsets. *J Allergy Clin Immunol* 123, 758-762 (2009).

[162] Lightfoot,K. *et al.* Does hepatitis GB virus-C infection cause hepatocellular carcinoma in black Africans? *Hepatology* 26, 740-742 (1997).

[163] Lin,H.H., Kao,J.H., Chen,P.J. & Chen,D.S. Mechanism of vertical transmission of hepatitis G. *Lancet* 347, 1116 (1996).

[164] Linnen,J. *et al.* Molecular cloning and disease association of hepatitis G virus: a transfusion-transmissible agent. *Science* 271, 505-508 (1996).

[165] liu,H. *et al.* The Vif protein of human and simian immunodeficiency viruses is packaged into virions and associates with viral core structures. *J Virol* 69, 7630-7638 (1995).

[166] Liu,H.F., Muyembe-Tamfum,J.J., Dahan,K., Desmyter,J. & Goubau,P. High prevalence of GB virus C/hepatitis G virus in Kinshasa. *J Med Virol* 60, 159-165 (2000).

[167] Lo,S.Y. *et al.* Detection of serologic responses to GB virus C/hepatitis G virus infection. *Int J Infect Dis* 6, 223-227 (2002).

[168] Lou,S. *et al.* Immunoassays to study prevalence of antibody against GB virus C in blood donors. *J Virol Methods* 68, 45-55 (1997).

[169] Lu,Y.L., Spearman,P. & Ratner,L. HIV-1 viral protein R localization in infected cells and virions. *J Virol* 67, 6542-6550 (1993).

[170] Lusso,P. *et al.* Growth of macrophage-tropic and primary human immunodeficiency virus type 1 (HIV-1) isolates in a unique CD4+ T-cell clone (PM1): failure to downregulate CD4 and to interfere with cell-line-tropic HIV-1. *J Virol* 69, 3712-3720 (1995).

[171] Macalalad,A.R. & Snydman,D.R. GB virus C and mortality from HIV infection. *N Engl J Med* 346, 377-379 (2002).

[172] Maddon,P.J. *et al.* The T4 gene encodes the AIDS virus receptor and is expressed in the immune system and the brain. *Cell* 47, 333-348 (1986).

[173] Madejon,A. *et al.* GB virus C RNA in serum, liver, and peripheral blood mononuclear cells from patients with chronic hepatitis B, C, and D. *Gastroenterology* 113, 573-578 (1997).

[174] Mansouritorghabeh,H. Detection of HGV E2 antibody in blood donors. *Int J Infect Dis* 12, 445-446 (2008).

[175] Mariani,R. *et al.* CCR2-64I polymorphism is not associated with altered CCR5 expression or coreceptor function. *J Virol* 73, 2450-2459 (1999).

[176] Martin,S.J. *et al.* Immunization of human HIV-seronegative volunteers with recombinant p17/p24:Ty virus-like particles elicits HIV-1 p24-specific cellular and humoral immune responses. *AIDS* 7, 1315-1323 (1993).

[177] Masur,H. et al. CD4 counts as predictors of opportunistic pneumonias in HIV infection. Ann Intern Med 111, 223-231 (1989).

[178] Matyas,G.R., Beck,Z., Karasavvas,N. & Alving,C.R. Lipid binding properties of 4E10, 2F5, and WR304 monoclonal antibodies that neutralize HIV-1. Biochim Biophys Acta 1788, 660-665 (2009).

[179] Matyas,G.R. et al. Neutralizing antibodies induced by liposomal HIV-1 glycoprotein 41 peptide simultaneously bind to both the 2F5 or 4E10 epitope and lipid epitopes. AIDS 23, 2069-2077 (2009).

[180] Mazzini,S. et al. 3D-Structure of the interior fusion peptide of HGV/GBV-C by 1H NMR, CD and molecular dynamics studies. Arch Biochem Biophys 465, 187-196 (2007).

[181] McCune,J.M. et al. Endoproteolytic cleavage of gp160 is required for the activation of human immunodeficiency virus. Cell 53, 55-67 (1988).

[182] McCutchan,F.E. Understanding the genetic diversity of HIV-1. AIDS 14 Suppl 3, S31-S44 (2000).

[183] McCutchan,F.E. Global epidemiology of HIV. J Med Virol 78 Suppl 1, S7-S12 (2006).

[184] McLinden,J.H. et al. Characterization of an immunodominant antigenic site on GB virus C glycoprotein E2 that is involved in cell binding. J Virol 80, 12131-12140 (2006).

[185] McLinden,J.H., Stapleton,J.T., Chang,Q. & Xiang,J. Expression of the dengue virus type 2 NS5 protein in a CD4(+) T cell line inhibits HIV replication. J Infect Dis 198, 860-863 (2008).

[186] Michalak,J.P. et al. Characterization of truncated forms of hepatitis C virus glycoproteins. J Gen Virol 78, 2299-2306 (1997).

[187] Moenkemeyer,M., Schmidt,R.E., Wedemeyer,H., Tillmann,H.L. & Heiken,H. GBV-C coinfection is negatively correlated to Fas expression and Fas-mediated apoptosis in HIV-1 infected patients. J Med Virol 80, 1933-1940 (2008).

[188] Monath,T.P. et al. Single mutation in the flavivirus envelope protein hinge region increases neurovirulence for mice and monkeys but decreases viscerotropism for monkeys: relevance to development and safety testing of live, attenuated vaccines. J Virol 76, 1932-1943 (2002).

[189] Montagnier L et al. A new human T-lymphotropic retrovirus: Characterization and possible role in lymphadenopathy and acquired immune deficiency syndromes. Book (1984).

[190] Montero,M., van Houten,N.E., Wang,X. & Scott,J.K. The membrane-proximal external region of the HIV type 1 envelope: dominant site of antibody neutralization and target for vaccine design. Microbiol Mol Biol Rev 72, 54-84 (2008).

[191] Moody,M.A. et al. Anti-phospholipid human monoclonal antibodies inhibit CCR5-tropic HIV-1 and induce beta-chemokines. J Exp Med 207, 763-776 (2010).

[192] Moore,P.S. et al. Primary characterization of a herpesvirus agent associated with Kaposi's sarcomae. J Virol 70, 549-558 (1996).

[193] Mueller,R. Untersuchung zur GBV-C vermittelten HIV-Hemmung in Herpesvirus saimiri transformierten Lymphozyten. Diploma thesis (2006).

[194] Muerhoff,A.S., Dawson,G.J. & Desai,S.M. A previously unrecognized sixth genotype of GB virus C revealed by analysis of 5'-untranslated region sequences. J Med Virol 78, 105-111 (2006).

[195] Nattermann,J. et al. Regulation of CC chemokine receptor 5 in hepatitis G virus infection. AIDS 17, 1457-1462 (2003).

[196] Ni,L., Gao,G.F. & Tien,P. Rational design of highly potent HIV-1 fusion inhibitory proteins: implication for developing antiviral therapeutics. Biochem Biophys Res Commun 332, 831-836 (2005).

[197] NIAID. New Discoveries Energize the HIV Vaccine Field: Report from AIDS Vaccine 2008 Meeting. (2009).

[198] Nielsen,C., Pedersen,C., Lundgren,J.D. & Gerstoft,J. Biological properties of HIV isolates in primary HIV infection: consequences for the subsequent course of infection. AIDS 7, 1035-1040 (1993).

[199] Nishiya,A.S. et al. Genotype distribution of the GB virus C in citizens of Sao Paulo City, Brazil. Rev Inst Med Trop Sao Paulo 45, 213-216 (2003).

[200] Noguchi,S. et al. GB virus C (GBV-C)/hepatitis G virus (HGV) infection in a hepatitis C virus hyper-endemic area in Japan. Hepatology Research 7, 149-158 (1997).

[201] Nordbo,S.A., Krokstad,S., Winge,P., Skjeldestad,F.E. & Dalen,A.B. Prevalence of GB virus C (also called hepatitis G virus) markers in Norwegian blood donors. J Clin Microbiol 38, 2584-2590 (2000).

[202] Northfield,J.W., Harcourt,G., Lucas,M. & Klenerman,P. Immunology of viral co-infections with HIV. Arch. Immunol Ther Exp 53, 3-12 (2005).

[203] Nunnari,G., Nigro,L., Palermo,F., Attanasio,M., Berger,A. Doerr,H.W., Pomerantz,R.J. & Cacopardo,B. Slower progression of HIV-1 infection in persons with GB virus C co-infection correlates with an intact T-helper 1 cytokine profile. Ann Intern Med 2003 139, 26-30 (2003).

[204] Ono,A., Ablan,S.D., Lockett,S.J., Nagashima,K. & Freed,E.O. Phosphatidylinositol (4,5) bisphosphate regulates HIV-1 Gag targeting to the plasma membrane. Proc Natl Acad Sci USA 101, 14889-14894 (2004).

[205] Oshima,M. et al. cDNA clones of Japanese hepatitis C virus genomes derived from a single patient show sequence heterogeneity. J Gen Virol 72, 2805-2809 (1991).

[206] Osmanov,S., Pattou,C., Walker,N., Schwardlander,B. & Esparza,J. Estimated global distribution and regional spread of HIV-1 genetic subtypes in the year 2000. J Acquir Immune Defic Syndr 29, 184-190 (2002).

[207] Ott,D.E. Cellular proteins in HIV virions. Rev Med Virol 7, 167-180 (1997).

[208] Ott,D.E. et al. Cytoskeletal proteins inside human immunodeficiency virus type 1 virions. J Virol 70, 7734-7743 (1996).

[209] Otto,C., Puffer,B.A., Pohlmann,S., Doms,R.W. & Kirchhoff,F. Mutations in the C3 region of human and simian immunodeficiency virus envelope have differential effects on viral infectivity, replication, and CD4-dependency. Virology 315, 292-302 (2003).

[210] Oubina,J.R. et al. Genetic diversity of GBV-C/HGV strains among HIV infected-IVDU and blood donors from Buenos Aires, Argentina. Virus Res 65, 121-129 (1999).

[211] Pacheco-Castro,A. et al. Herpesvirus saimiri immortalization of alpha beta and gamma delta human T-lineage cells derived from CD34+ intrathymic precursors in vitro. Int Immunol 8, 1797-1805 (1996).

[212] Panda,S.K., Panigrahi,A.K., Dasarathy,S. & Acharya,S.K. Hepatitis G virus in India. Lancet 348, 1319 (1996).

[213] Pandori,M.W. et al. Producer-cell modification of HIV type 1: Nef is a virion protein. J Virol 70, 4283-4290 (1996).

[214] Pantaleo,G. et al. Major expansion of CD8+ T cells with a predominant V beta usage during the primary immune response to HIV. Nature 370, 463-467 (1994).

[215] Pantophlet,R. Neutralizing antibodies, Mucosal immunology: A Summary. Rapporteur Session AIDS Vaccine 2008: B cell immunology, (2008).

[216] Pavesi,A. Detection of signature sequences in overlapping genes and prediction of a novel overlapping gene in hepatitis G virus. J Mol Evol 50, 284-295 (2000).

[217] Pavlova,B.G. et al. Association of GB virus C (GBV-C)/hepatitis G virus (HGV) with haematological diseases of different malignant potential. J Med Virol 57, 361-366 (1999).

[218] Peeters M. Recombinant HIV Sequences: Their Role in the Global Epidemic. 2000.

[219] Pereira,L.A., Bentley,K., Peeters,A., Churchill,M.J. & Deacon,N.J. A compilation of cellular transcription factor interactions with the HIV-1 LTR promoter. Nucleic Acids Res 28, 663-668 (2000).

[220] Perrin,L. Primary HIV infection. *Antivir Ther* 4 Suppl 3, 13-18 (1999).

[221] Pileri,P. et al. Binding of hepatitis C virus to CD81. *Science* 282, 938-941 (1998).

[222] Pinto,L.A. et al. Influenza virus-stimulated generation of anti-HIV activity after influenza vaccination in HIV-infected individuals and healthy control subjects. *J Infect Dis* 183, 1000-1008 (2001).

[223] Pinto,L.A. et al. Inhibition of human immunodeficiency virus type 1 replication prior to reverse transcription by influenza virus stimulation. *J Virol* 74, 4505-4511 (2000).

[224] Pomerantz,R.J. & Nunnari,G. HIV and GB virus C--can two viruses be better than one? *N Engl J Med* 350, 963-5 (2004).

[225] Platt,E.J., Wehrly,K., Kuhmann,S.E., Chesebro,B. & Kabat,D. Effects of CCR5 and CD4 cell surface concentrations on infections by macrophagetropic isolates of human immunodeficiency virus type 1. *J Virol* 72, 2855-2864 (1997).

[226] Price,D.A. et al. Positive selection of HIV-1 cytotoxic T lymphocyte escape variants during primary infection. *Proc Natl Acad Sci USA* 94, 1890-1895 (1997).

[227] Puck,T.T., Cieciura,S.J. & Robinson,A. Genetics of somatic mammalian cells. III. Long-term cultivation of euploid cells from human and animal subjects. *J Exp Med* 108, 945-956 (1958).

[228] Purcell,R.H. The discovery of the hepatitis viruses. *Gastroenterology* 104, 955-963 (1993).

[229] Quinn,T.C. Global burden of the HIV pandemic. *Lancet* 348, 99-106 (1996).

[230] Randell,P. & Moyle,G. Antiretroviral therapy with heart. *Am J Ther* 16, 579-584 (2009).

[231] Reed,K.E. & Rice,C.M. Overview of hepatitis C virus genome structure, polyprotein processing, and protein properties. *Curr Top Microbiol Immunol* 242, 55-84 (2000).

[232] Rendina,D. et al. HCV and GBV-c/HGV infection in HIV positive patients in southern Italy. *Eur J Epidemiol.* 17, 801-807 (2001).

[233] Richter,M. Entwicklung Antigen-basierter Capture ELISA zum serodiagnostischen Nachweis GBV-C spezifischer Antikörper. Diploma thesis (2009).

[234] Rio,D.C., Clark,S.G. & Tjian,R. A mammalian host-vector system that regulates expression and amplification of transfected genes by temperature induction. *Science* 227, 23-28 (1985).

[235] Robertson,D.L. et al. HIV-1 nomenclature proposal. *Science* 288, 55-56 (2000).

[236] Rothwangl,K.B. & Rong,L. Analysis of a conserved RGE/RGD motif in HCV E2 in mediating entry. *Virol J* 6, 12 (2009).

[237] Roy,A., Kucukural,A. & Zhang,Y. I-TASSER: a unified platform for automated protein structure and function prediction. *Nat. Protoc* 5, 725-738 (2010).

[238] Ruel,T.D. et al. HIV RNA suppression among HIV-infected Ugandan children with measles. *J Acquir Immune Defic Syndr* 48, 225-227 (2008).

[239] Saad,J.S. et al. Point mutations in the HIV-1 matrix protein turn off the myristyl switch. *J Mol Biol* 366, 574-585 (2007).

[240] Sabin,C.A. et al. Effect of coinfection with hepatitis G virus on HIV disease progression in hemophilic men. *J Acquir Immune Defic Syndr Hum Retrovirol* 19, 546-548 (1998).

[241] Salmon-Ceron,D. et al. Safety and immunogenicity of a recombinant HIV type 1 glycoprotein 160 boosted by a V3 synthetic peptide in HIV-negative volunteers. *AIDS Res Hum Retroviruses* 11, 1479-1486 (1995).

[242] Salter,R.D. Genes regulating HLA class I antigen expression in T-B lymphoblast hybrids. *Immunogenetics* 21, 235-246 (1985).

[243] Sanger,F., Coulson,A.R., Barrell,B.G., Smith,A.J. & Roe,B.A. Cloning in single-stranded bacteriophage as an aid to rapid DNA sequencing. *J Mol Biol* 143, 161-178 (1980).

[244] Sanger,F., Nicklen,S. & Coulson,A.R. DNA sequencing with chain-terminating inhibitors. *Proc Natl Acad Sci USA* 74, 5463-5467 (1977).

[245] Sathar,M., Soni,P. & York,D. GB virus C/hepatitis G virus (GBV-C/HGV): still looking for a disease. *Int J Exp Pathol* 81, 305-322 (2000).

[246] Sawai,E.T. et al. Human immunodeficiency virus type 1 Nef associates with a cellular serine kinase in T lymphocytes. *Proc Natl Acad Sci USA* 91, 1539-1543 (1994).

[247] Scarselli,E. et al. The human scavenger receptor class B type I is a novel candidate receptor for the hepatitis C virus. *EMBO J* 21, 5017-5025 (2002).

[248] Schacker,T.W., Hughes,J.P., Shea,T., Coombs,R.W. & Corey,L. Biological and virologic characteristics of primary HIV infection. *Ann Intern Med* 128, 613-620 (1998).

[249] Schaluder,G.G. et al. Molecular and serologic analysis in the transmission of the GB hepatitis agents. *J Med Virol* 46, 81-90 (1995).

[250] Schiefer,H.G. The orientation of serologically active phospholipids in mitochondrial membranes, I. *Hoppe Seylers Z Physiol Chem* 354, 722-724 (1973).

[251] Schmidt,B., Korn,K. & Fleckenstein,B. Molecular evidence for transmission of hepatitis G virus by blood transfusion. *Lancet* 347, 909 (1996).

[252] Schmolke,S., Tacke,M., Schmitt,U., Engel,A.M. & Ofenloch-Haehnle,B. Identification of hepatitis G virus particles in human serum by E2-specific monodonal antibodies generated by DNA immunization. *J Virol* 72, 4541-4545 (1998).

[253] Schneider,U. & Schwenk,H.U. Characterization of "T" and "non-T" cell lines established from children with acute lymphoblastic leukemia and non-Hodgkin lymphoma after leukemic transformation. *Haematol Blood Transfus* 20, 265-269 (1977).

[254] Schreier,E., Hohne,M., Kunkel,U., Berg,T. & Hopf,U. Hepatitis GBV-C sequences in patients infected with HCV contaminated anti-D immunoglobulin and among i.v. drug users in Germany. *Hepatology* 25, 385-389 (1996).

[255] Schriebl,K. et al. Biochemical characterization of rhEpo-Fc fusion protein expressed in CHO cells. *Protein Expr Purif* 49, 265-275 (2006).

[256] Schwartz,D.H. et al. Induction of HIV-1-neutralising and syncytium-inhibiting antibodies in uninfected recipients of HIV-1IIIB rgp120 subunit vaccine. *Lancet* 342, 69-73 (1993).

[257] Sealy,R. et al. Preclinical and clinical development of a multi-envelope, DNA-virus-protein (D-V-P) HIV-1 vaccine. *Int Rev Immunol* 28, 49-68 (2009).

[258] Sharp,P.M. et al. The origins of AIDS viruses: where and when? *Philos Trans R Soc Lond B Biol Sci* 356, 867-876 (2001).

[259] Sharp,P.M., Robertson,D.L. & Hahn,B.H. Cross-species transmission and recombination of 'AIDS' viruses. *Philos Trans R Soc Lond B Biol Sci* 349, 41-47 (1995).

[260] Shepard,R.N. et al. Quantitation of HIV type 1 RNA in different biological compartments. *J Clin Microbiol* 38, 1414-1418 (2000).

[261] Simons,J.N., Desai,S.M. & Mushahwar,I.K. The GB viruses. *Curr Top Microbiol Immunol* 242, 341-375 (2000).

[262] Simons,J.N., Desai,S.M., Schultz,D.E., Lemon,S.M. & Mushahwar,I.K. Translation initiation in GB viruses A and C: evidence for internal ribosome entry and implications for genome organization. *J Virol* 70, 6126-6135 (1996).

[263] Simons,J.N. Isolation of novel virus-like sequences associated with human hepatitis. *Nat Med* 1, 564-569 (1995).

[264] Simons,J.N. et al. Identification of two flavivirus-like genomes in the GB hepatitis agent. *Proc Natl Acad Sci USA* 92, 3401-3405 (1995).

[265] Smith,D.B. et al. Phylogenetic analysis of GBV-C/hepatitis G virus. *J Gen Virol* 81, 769-780 (2000).

[266] Sodroski,J. et al. A second post-transcriptional trans-activator gene required for HTLV-III replication. *Nature* 321, 412-417 (1986).

[267] Stapleton,J.T. & Chaloner,K. GB virus C infection and non-Hodgkin lymphoma: important to know but the jury is out. *Int J Cancer* (2010).

[268] Stark,K. et al. Detection of the hepatitis G virus genome among injecting drug users, homosexual and bisexual men, and blood donors. *J Infect Dis* 174, 1320-1323 (1996).

[269] Stitz,J. et al. Lentiviral vectors pseudotyped with envelope glycoproteins derived from gibbon ape leukemia virus and murine leukemia virus 10A1. *Virology* 273, 16-20 (2000).

[270] Stroud,J.C., Oltman,A., Han,A., Bates,D.L. & Chen,L. Structural basis of HIV-1 activation by NF-kappaB--a higher-order complex of p50:RelA bound to the HIV-1 LTR. *J Mol Biol* 393, 98-112 (2009).

[271] Subbramanian,R.A. & Cohen,E.A. Molecular biology of the HIV accessory proteins. *J Virol* 68, 6831-6835 (1994).

[272] Sun,J. et al. SEPPA: a computational server for spatial epitope prediction of protein antigens. *Nucleic Acids Res.* 37, W612-W616 (2009).

[273] Sun,Z.Y. et al. HIV-1 broadly neutralizing antibody extracts its epitope from a kinked gp41 ectodomain region on the viral membrane. *Immunity* 28, 52-63 (2008).

[274] Superti,F. et al. Entry pathway of vesicular stomatitis virus into different host cells. *J Gen Virol* 68, 387-399 (1987).

[275] Swanson,M.D., Winter,H.C., Goldstein,I.J. & Markovitz,D.M. A lectin isolated from bananas is a potent inhibitor of HIV replication. *J Biol Chem* 285, 8646-8655 (2010).

[276] Tabor,E., Seeff,L.B. & Gerety,R.J. Lack of susceptibility of marmosets to human non-A, non-B hepatitis. *J Infect Dis* 140, 794-797 (1979).

[277] Tacke,M. et al. Detection of antibodies to a putative hepatitis G virus envelope protein. *Lancet* 349, 318-320 (1997).

[278] Tacke,M. et al. Humoral immune response to the E2 protein of hepatitis G virus is associated with long-term recovery from infection and reveals a high frequency of hepatitis G virus exposure among healthy blood donors. *Hepatology* 26, 1626-1633 (1997).

[279] Tagger,A. et al. Prevalence of GB virus-C/hepatitis G virus infection in patients with cryptogenic chronic liver disease and in patients with primary biliary cirrhosis or Wilson's disease. *Am J Gastroenterol* 94, 484-488 (1999).

[280] Takahashi,K. et al. Characterization of GBV-C/HGV viral genome: comparison among different isolates for a ~2 kb-sequence that covers entire E1 and most of 5'UTR and E2. *International Hepatology Communications* 6, 253-263 (1997).

[281] Tan,D. et al. Analysis of hepatitis G virus (HGV) RNA, antibody to HGV envelope protein, and risk factors for blood donors coinfected with HGV and hepatitis C virus. *J Infect Dis* 179, 1055-1061 (1999).

[282] Tanaka,Y. et al. African origin of GB virus C/hepatitis G virus. *FEBS Lett* 423, 143-148 (1998).

[283] Tao,W. et al. A single point mutation in E2 enhances hepatitis C virus infectivity and alters lipoprotein association of viral particles. *Virology* 395, 67-76 (2009).

[284] Thio,C.L. Hepatitis B and human immunodeficiency virus coinfection. *Hepatology* 49, S138-S145 (2009).

[285] Thomas,D.L. The challenge of hepatitis C in the HIV-infected person. *Annu Rev Med* 59, 473-485 (2008).

[286] Thomas,D.L. et al. Association of antibody to GB virus C (hepatitis G virus) with viral clearance and protection from reinfection. *J Infect Dis* 177, 539-542 (1998).

[287] Tillmann,H.L. et al. Infection with GB virus C and reduced mortality among HIV-infected patients. *N Engl J Med* 345, 715-724 (2001).

[288] Tillmann,H.L. et al. Antibodies against the GB virus C envelope 2 protein before liver transplantation protect against GB virus C de novo infection. *Hepatology* 28, 379-384 (1998).

[289] Toscano,M.G. et al. Efficient lentiviral transduction of Herpesvirus saimiri immortalized T cells as a model for gene therapy in primary immunodeficiencies. *Gene Ther* 11, 956-961 (2004).

[290] Tucker,T.J., Louw,S.J., Robson,S.C., Isaacs,S. & Kirsch,R.E. High prevalence of GBV-C hepatitis G virus infection in a rural South African population. *J Med Virol* 53, 225-228 (1997).

[291] Tucker,T.J. & Smuts,H.E. GBV-C/HGV genotypes: proposed nomenclature for genotypes 1-5. *J Med Virol.* 62, 82-83 (2000).

[292] Tucker,T.J. et al. Evidence that the GBV-C/hepatitis G virus is primarily a lymphotropic virus. *J Med Virol* 61, 52-58 (2000).

[293] Tuveri,R. et al. Prevalence and genetic variants of hepatitis GB-C/HG and TT viruses in Gabon, equatorial Africa. *Am J Trop Med Hyg* 63, 192-198 (2000).

[294] UNAIDS and WHO. AIDS epidemic update: December 2009. Report (2009).

[295] Unutmaz,D., KewalRamani,V.N. & Littman,D.R. G protein-coupled receptors in HIV and SIV entry: new perspectives on lentivirus-host interactions. *Semin Immunol* 10, 225-236 (1998).

[296] Urlaub,G. & Chasin,L.A. Isolation of Chinese hamster cell mutants deficient in dihydrofolate reductase activity. *Proc Natl Acad Sci USA* 77, 4216-4220 (1980).

[297] van Asten,L. & Prins,M. Infection with concurrent multiple hepatitis C virus genotypes is associated with faster HIV disease progression. *AIDS* 18, 2319-2324 (2004).

[298] van,M.G., Voelker,D.R. & Feigenson,G.W. Membrane lipids: where they are and how they behave. *Nat Rev Mol Cell Biol* 9, 112-124 (2008).

[299] Vella,C., Zheng,N.N., Easterbrook,P. & Daniels,R.S. Herpesvirus saimiri-immortalized human lymphocytes: novel hosts for analyzing HIV type 1 in vitro neutralization. *AIDS Res Hum Retroviruses* 18, 933-946 (2002).

[300] Venter,A. Hepatitis G virus slows HIV. *Trends Microbiol.* 9, 470 (2001).

[301] Viazov,S. et al. Transmission of GBV-C/HGV from drug-addicted mothers to their babies. *J Hepatol* 27, 85-90 (1997).

[302] Vogt,M. et al. Prevalence and clinical role of GBV-C infection after cardiac surgery in childhood: A study on 414 patients. *J Infect* (2005).

[303] Watt,G. et al. HIV-1 suppression during acute scrub-typhus infection. *Lancet* 356, 475-479 (2000).

[304] Wei,X. et al. Antibody neutralization and escape by HIV-1. *Nature* 422, 307-312 (2003).

[305] Weiner,A.J. et al. Variable and hypervariable domains are found in the regions of HCV corresponding to the flavivirus envelope and NS1 proteins and the pestivirus envelope glycoproteins. *Virology* 180, 842-848 (1991).

[306] Weiss,A., Wiskocil,R.L. & Stobo,J.D. The role of T3 surface molecules in the activation of human T cells: a two-stimulus requirement for IL 2 production reflects events occurring at a pre-translational level. *J Immunol* 133, 123-128 (1984).

[307] Weiss,C.D., Levy,J.A. & White,J.M. Oligomeric organization of gp120 on infectious HIV-1 particles. *J Virol* 64, 5674-5677 (1990).

[308] Williams,C.F. et al. Persistent GB virus C infection and survival in HIV-infected men. *N Engl J Med* 350, 981-990 (2004).

[309] Wiwanitkit,V. Hepatitis G virus RNA positivity among the voluntary blood donors: a summary. *Ann Hepatol* 4, 43-46 (2005).

[310] Wong,K., Li,X. & Ma,Y. Paraformaldehyde induces elevation of intracellular calcium and phosphatidylserine externalization in platelets. *Thromb Res* 117, 537-542 (2006).

[311] Wu,L., Martin,T.D., Carrington,M. & KewalRamani,V.N. Raji B cells, misidentified as THP-1 cells, stimulate DC-SIGN-mediated HIV transmission. *Virology* 318, 17-23 (2004).

[312] Xiang,J. *et al.* Inhibition of HIV-1 replication by GB virus C infection through increases in RANTES, MIP-1alpha, MIP-1beta, and SDF-1. *Lancet* 363, 2040-2046 (2004).

[313] Xiang,J. *et al.* Characterization of hepatitis G virus (GB-C virus) particles: evidence for a nucleocapsid and expression of sequences upstream of the E1 protein. *J Virol* 72, 2738-2744 (1998).

[314] Xiang,J., McLinden,J.H., Chang,Q., Jordan,E.L. & Stapleton,J.T. Characterization of a peptide domain within the GB virus C NS5A phosphoprotein that inhibits HIV replication. *PLoS ONE* 3, e2580 (2008).

[315] Xiang,J., McLinden,J.H., Chang,Q., Kaufman,T.M. & Stapleton,J.T. An 85-aa segment of the GB virus type C NS5A phosphoprotein inhibits HIV-1 replication in CD4+ Jurkat T cells. *Proc Natl Acad Sci USA* 103, 15570-15575 (2006).

[316] Xiang,J. *et al.* Viruses within the Flaviviridae decrease CD4 expression and inhibit HIV replication in human CD4+ cells. *J Immunol* 183, 7860-7869 (2009).

[317] Xiang,J. *et al.* Effect of coinfection with GB virus C on survival among patients with HIV infection. *N Engl J Med* 345, 707-714 (2001).

[318] Xiang,J., Wunschmann,S., Schmidt,W., Shao,J. & Stapleton,J.T. Full-length GB virus C (Hepatitis G virus) RNA transcripts are infectious in primary CD4-positive T cells. *J Virol* 74, 9125-9133 (2000).

[319] Yasumura,Y. & Kawakita,Y. Studies on SV40 in tissue culture-preliminary step for cancer research in vitro. *Jpn J Clin Med* 21, 1201-1215 (1963).

[320] Yeo,A.E. *et al.* Effect of hepatitis G virus infection on progression of HIV infection in patients with hemophilia. Multicenter Hemophilia Cohort Study. *Ann Intern Med* 132, 959-963 (2000).

[321] Zachowski,A. Phospholipids in animal eukaryotic membranes: transverse asymmetry and movement. *Biochem J* 294, 1-14 (1993).

[322] Zhang,W., Chaloner,K., Tillmann,H.L., Williams,C.F., Stapleton,J.T. Effect of early and late GB virus C viraemia on survival of HIV-infected individuals: a meta-analysis. *HIV Med* 7, 173-80 (2006).

[323] Zhang,Y. I-TASSER server for protein 3D structure prediction. *BMC Bioinformatics* 9, 40 (2008).

[324] Zhu,P. *et al.* Electron tomography analysis of envelope glycoprotein trimers on HIV and simian immunodeficiency virus virions. *Proc Natl Acad Sci USA* 100, 15812-15817 (2003).

[325] Zhu,P. *et al.* Distribution and three-dimensional structure of AIDS virus envelope spikes. *Nature* 441, 847-852 (2006).

[326] Zolla-Pazner,S., Gorny,M.K., Nyambi,P.N., VanCott,T.C. & Nadas,A. Immunotyping of human immunodeficiency virus type 1 (HIV): an approach to immunologic classification of HIV. *J Virol* 73, 4042-4051 (1999).

# 11. Publications

Some of the research was originally published in:

Jung, S., Knauer, O., Donhauser, N., Eichenmüller, M., Helm, M., Fleckenstein, B., Reil H. Inhibition of HIV strains by GB Virus C in cell culture can be mediated by CD4+ and CD8+ T-lymphocyte derived soluble factors. AIDS, 19 (12), 1267-72 (2005)

Jung, S., Eichenmueller, M., Donhauser, N., Neipel, F., Engel, A., Hess, G., Fleckenstein, B., Reil, H. HIV entry inhibition by the envelope 2 glycoprotein of GB Virus C. AIDS, 21 (5), 645-647 (2007).

Jochmann, R., Thurau, M., Jung, S., Hofmann, C., Naschberger, E., Kremmer, E., Harrer, T., Miller, M., Schaft, N., Stürzl, M. O-linked N-Acetylglucosaminylation of Sp1 Inhibits the Human Immunodeficiency Virus Type-1 Promoter. J Virol, 83 (8), 3704-18 (2009).

# 12. Acknowledgements

Though only my name appears on the cover of this dissertation, many people have contributed to this work. The writing of this dissertation has been one of the most significant academic challenges I have ever had to face. Many people have helped me stay sane through these difficult years. Without the support, patience and guidance of the following people, this work would not have been completed. It is to them that I owe my gratitude.

My deepest gratitude is due to my supervisors who assisted me with so much care and patience. I like to thank Prof. Bernhard Fleckenstein who undertook to act as my mentor despite his many other academic commitments and supervised my graduate work from the outset to the very end. Furthermore, I am deeply indebted to Dr. Dr. Heide Reil. I have been amazingly fortunate to have an advisor who gave me the freedom to explore on my own and at the same time the guidance to recover when my steps faltered. Her patience and support helped me overcome many crises and finish this dissertation. My thanks also go to Prof. Wolfgang Hillen for agreeing to serve as doctoral thesis supervisor.

Thanks to all the present and former lab members. I am grateful to Holger Wend and Norbert Donhauser, who participated on my projects and gave me a hand at sometimes unpleasant routines making my high throughput assays possible. I like to thanks Melanie Eichenmueller, Ralf Mueller, and Mandy Richter who suffered my supervision during their diploma thesis. Their dedicated and successful work had substantial impact on my doctoral thesis.

This work would not have been possible without the support of the staff of the clinical diagnostic department who answered questions, shared bench and equipment as soon as possible and performed assays where required. Many thanks to the central service for providing an excellent environment for my scientific research. Moreover, my sincere thanks also go to everyone else who supported me from time to time by collaborative behavior and valuable discussion along the way. I am indebted to my co-operation partners Prof. Hans L. Tillmann and Solveig Tenckhoff, Prof. Jack T. Stapelton, Dr. Jinhua Xiang, and Dr. Jim H. McLinden as well as Dr. Alfred M. Engel and Dr. Michael Tacke.

The best are kept for the last. Nobody has been more important to me in the pursuit of this project than the members of my family. This thesis is dedicated to my parents and my family for always supporting me, in many ways, all the way – through their love, their compassion and encouragement. Her unwavering faith and confidence in my abilities and in me is what has shaped me to be the person I am today. Very special thanks also to my friends who helped me reach the finish line. Notably Orsy, who always keep an eye on me, but also Wolf, Moni, Steffi, and Mandy for all the fun during the days holding pipettes and during the nights holding beers. Their support and care helped me overcome setbacks and stay focused on my graduate study and sane through these difficult years. I greatly value their friendship and I deeply appreciate their belief in me.

Finally, in a world where hard cash is at a premium, I thank the graduate training program Viruses of the Immune System of the German Research Foundation, the Academy of Sciences and Literature, the Competence Net Hepatitis as well as the Interdisciplinary Center for Clinical Research of the University Hospital Erlangen for generously funding.

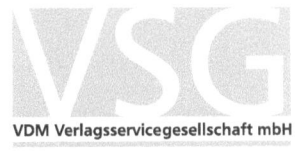

Die VDM Verlagsservicegesellschaft sucht für wissenschaftliche Verlage abgeschlossene und herausragende

## Dissertationen, Habilitationen, Diplomarbeiten, Master Theses, Magisterarbeiten usw.

für die kostenlose Publikation als Fachbuch.

Sie verfügen über eine Arbeit, die hohen inhaltlichen und formalen Ansprüchen genügt, und haben Interesse an einer honorarvergüteten Publikation?

Dann senden Sie bitte erste Informationen über sich und Ihre Arbeit per Email an *info@vdm-vsg.de*.

**Sie erhalten kurzfristig unser Feedback!**

VDM Verlagsservicegesellschaft mbH
Dudweiler Landstr. 99
D - 66123 Saarbrücken
Telefon +49 681 3720 174
Fax     +49 681 3720 1749
**www.vdm-vsg.de**

Die VDM Verlagsservicegesellschaft mbH vertritt

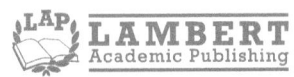
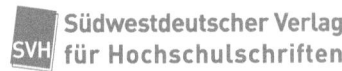

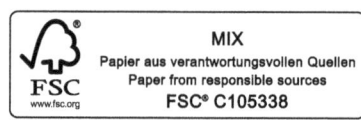

Printed by Books on Demand GmbH, Norderstedt / Germany